The Mediterranean Diet Cookbook 2021 for the Family:

Perfectly Portioned Recipes for Healthy Eating.

TABLE OF CONTENTS

INTRODUCTION

The principles of the Mediterranean diet are simple and easy to follow. You'll be pleased to discover that the Mediterranean diet is more about what you can and should eat than what you shouldn't eat.

Eat A Plant-Based Diet

Build your meals around vegetables, fresh fruits, beans, and legumes. These whole foods are central to the health benefits of the Mediterranean diet. They provide energy in the form of complex carbohydrates, antioxidants, vitamins, minerals, phytochemicals, and fiber. These nutrient-dense foods fill you up and keep you satisfied, thus helping to control your weight while providing disease-fighting nutrients.

Choose Whole Grains

Avoid refined grains like white flour and rice. Choose whole grains such as whole wheat, brown rice, oats, barley, corn, quinoa, farro, bulgur, millet, and so on, including whole grain breads, and pasta. Whole grains are higher in nutrients, including minerals, vitamins, and fiber.

Eat Foods That Contain Healthy Fats, Including Olives, Olive Oil, Nuts, And Seeds

Olive and olive oil are rich in heart-healthy monounsaturated fats and antioxidants. Add olives and olive oil to your pasta, salads, and stews, and have them as a snack. Nuts and seeds, such as almonds, cashews, pine nuts, hazelnuts, pistachios, pumpkin seeds, sesame seeds, and walnuts are also good sources of healthy fats. Avoid fats that are higher in saturated fats such as butter, cream, lard, or red meat. Completely avoid trans fats such as hydrogenated oils and margarine.

Eat Fish and Seafood

Eat fish and seafood such as tuna, crab, squid, shrimp, sea bass, sardines, salmon, octopus, mussels, herring, cod, clams, bream, and anchovies.

Limit Dairy, Cheese, And Yogurt

Moderation Is the Key

It's vital to keep portion sizes in check when consuming high calorie and high saturated fat foods like cheese, red meat, refined grains, and foods sweetened with refined sugar.

Take Time to Enjoy Life and Be Physically Active

The Mediterranean way of life is more relaxed than the typical American lifestyle. People in this coastal region take the time to enjoy meals with their families. They walk or bike to work instead of driving, and they take far more vacation time -all of which can reduce stress and contribute to good health.

On the Mediterranean diet, you need to consume:

At least 4 servings of fresh fruits and vegetables per day.

3 to 5 servings of whole grains per day.

4 to 6 servings of healthy fats per day.

At least 3 servings of fish and seafood per week.

Up to 7 servings of dairy products per week.

Up to one 5-ounce glass of red wine per day for women and two glasses per day for men.

3 to 5 servings (2 eggs) per week.

2 to 5 serving of poultry per week.

Up to 4 servings of sweets per week.

3 to 5 servings of red meat per month.

The Fundamentals Food

General guidelines of the Mediterranean diet are collected in the Mediterranean Diet Pyramid. It's accepted as the "gold standard" dietary plan that boosts your health. The pyramid was created in 1993 and made the Mediterranean diet popular. The pyramid was developed by Oldways Preservation and Exchange Trust, and Harvard School of Public Health. The pyramid reflects the social and cultural traditions of the Mediterranean lifestyle.

The base of the pyramid showcases the great importance of strong social connection, exercise, and sharing meals with your family and friends. When following the Mediterranean diet, you should prioritize exercises such as running and aerobics, and even small things like walking up the stairs and housework. One of the biggest sections of the Mediterranean Diet Pyramid is devoted to plant-based foods. Fruits and vegetables, beans, whole grains, olive oil, nuts, herbs, and spices are the most important components, so you should consume them daily. Eat fresh and seasonal food and avoid processed foods as much as possible.

Mediterranean Diet Pyramid

Whole Grains, Vegetables, And Fruits

They're an integral part of the Mediterranean diet plan. The grains you should add to your diet should be non-refined whole grains such as quinoa and brown rice. Vegetables can include green leafy vegetables such as kale, spinach, broccoli, Brussels sprouts, cauliflower, and carrots.

Olive Oil

Olive oil is a very important part of the Mediterranean diet and is much healthier than other vegetable oils such as canola or sunflower oil. Use olive oil with every dish and replace butter and margarine with olive oil. Consume an average of ½ cup per week.

Beans, Nuts, And Seeds

Beans, nuts, seeds, and lentils are a great source of protein. Use these ingredients as a substitute for red meat where possible. They provide a more filling, more affordable, and healthier source of protein compared to red meats.

Spices

Use herbs and spices to flavor food instead of sodium-rich table salt. Get creative when flavoring food by combining fresh herbs with olive oil to marinade your food. Season dishes with fresh cracked black pepper for extra spiciness.

Fish and Seafood

The omega-3 oils found in fish is required for healthy brain development, and it helps reduce the risk of cardiovascular disease with regular consumption.

Poultry, Eggs, Cheese, And Yogurt

Include poultry, eggs, cheese, and yogurt in your daily diet. Always focus on moderate consumption of any dairy products and monitor their effects on you.

Meats

Red meat should be kept to a minimum, as it isn't the healthiest diet option and can be substituted with legumes, bean, and seeds. When you do eat red meat, try to eat grass fed, organic red meat and keep it to a minimal amount of servings per week.

Red Wine

Many studies have shown that one glass of red wine per day can have multiple health benefits. The Mediterranean diet recommends enjoying one glass of red wine. Remember, more than two glasses can be detrimental to your health.

Physical Activity and Social Interaction

The Mediterranean lifestyle includes moderate amounts of daily physical activity and social interaction. Mediterranean's walk or cycle to work and lead very active lifestyles. Meals are also enjoyed as a family and are eaten over a longer period of time with plenty of conversation and laughs in between. If you can't walk or bike to work, try to take short walks when home and engage in as much physical activity -such as taking the stairs instead of the elevator- during your normal day as possible, Sit down at breakfast, lunch, and dinner and take time to savor your food. Try to taste every bite and identify the ingredients in each bite. Use dinnertime to talk to your family and discuss everyone's day, some goals for the week, your hobbies, and anything interesting you may have seen or heard that day.

BREAKFAST RECIPES

1. Pear and Mango Smoothie

Preparation time: 5 minutes

Cooking time: 0 minutes

Servings: 1

INGREDIENTS:

- 1 ripe mango, cored and chopped
- ½ mango, peeled, pitted and chopped
- 1 cup kale, chopped
- ½ cup plain Greek yogurt
- 2 ice cubes

DIRECTIONS:

1. Add pear, mango, yogurt, kale, and mango to a blender and puree. Add ice and blend until you have a smooth texture. Serve and enjoy!

NUTRITION: Calories: 293 Fat: 8g Carbohydrates: 53g Protein: 8g

2. Eggplant Salad

Preparation time: 20 minutes

Cooking time: 15 minutes

Servings: 8

INGREDIENTS:

- 1 large eggplant, washed and cubed
- 1 tomato, seeded and chopped
- 1 small onion, diced
- 2 tablespoons parsley, chopped
- 2 tablespoons extra virgin olive oil
- 2 tablespoons distilled white vinegar
- ½ cup feta cheese, crumbled
- Salt as needed

DIRECTIONS:

1. Pre-heat your outdoor grill to medium-high. Pierce the eggplant a few times using a knife/fork. Cook the eggplants on your grill for about 15 minutes until they are charred.
2. Keep it on the side and allow them to cool. Remove the skin from the eggplant and dice the pulp. Transfer the pulp to a mixing bowl and add parsley, onion, tomato, olive oil, feta cheese and vinegar.
3. Mix well and chill for 1 hour. Season with salt and enjoy!

NUTRITION: Calories: 99 Fat: 7g Carbohydrates: 7g Protein: 3.4g

3. Artichoke Frittata

Preparation time: 5 minutes

Cooking time: 10 minutes

Servings: 4

INGREDIENTS:

- 8 large eggs

- ¼ cup Asiago cheese, grated
- 1 tablespoon fresh basil, chopped
- 1 teaspoon fresh oregano, chopped
- Pinch of salt
- 1 teaspoon extra virgin olive oil
- 1 teaspoon garlic, minced
- 1 cup canned artichokes, drained
- 1 tomato, chopped

DIRECTIONS:

1. Pre-heat your oven to broil. Take a medium bowl and whisk in eggs, Asiago cheese, oregano, basil, sea salt and pepper. Blend in a bowl.
2. Place a large ovenproof skillet over medium-high heat and add olive oil. Add garlic and sauté for 1 minute. Remove skillet from heat and pour in egg mix.
3. Return skillet to heat and sprinkle artichoke hearts and tomato over eggs. Cook frittata without stirring for 8 minutes.
4. Place skillet under the broiler for 1 minute until the top is lightly browned. Cut frittata into 4 pieces and serve. Enjoy!

NUTRITION: Calories: 199 Fat: 13g Carbohydrates: 5g Protein: 16g

4. Full Eggs in a Squash

Preparation time: 15 minutes
Cooking time: 20 minutes
Servings: 5

INGREDIENTS:

- 2 acorn squash
- 6 whole eggs
- 2 tablespoons extra virgin olive oil
- Salt and pepper as needed
- 5-6 pitted dates
- 8 walnut halves
- A fresh bunch of parsley

DIRECTIONS:

1. Pre-heat your oven to 375 degrees Fahrenheit. Slice squash crosswise and prepare 3 slices with holes. While slicing the squash, make sure that each slice has a measurement of ¾ inch thickness.

2. Remove the seeds from the slices. Take a baking sheet and line it with parchment paper. Transfer the slices to your baking sheet and season them with salt and pepper.

3. Bake in your oven for 20 minutes. Chop the walnuts and dates on your cutting board. Take the baking dish out of the oven and drizzle slices with olive oil.

4. Crack an egg into each of the holes in the slices and season with pepper and salt. Sprinkle the chopped walnuts on top. Bake for 10 minutes more. Garnish with parsley and add maple syrup.

NUTRITION: Calories: 198 Fat: 12g Carbohydrates: 17g Protein: 8g

5. Barley Porridge

Preparation time: 5 minutes

Cooking time: 25 minutes

Servings: 4

INGREDIENTS:

- 1 cup barley
- 1 cup wheat berries
- 2 cups unsweetened almond milk
- 2 cups water
- ½ cup blueberries
- ½ cup pomegranate seeds
- ½ cup hazelnuts, toasted and chopped
- ¼ cup honey

DIRECTIONS:

1. Take a medium saucepan and place it over medium-high heat. Place barley, almond milk, wheat berries, water and bring to a boil. Reduce the heat to low and simmer for 25 minutes.
2. Divide amongst serving bowls and top each serving with 2 tablespoons blueberries, 2 tablespoons pomegranate seeds, 2 tablespoons hazelnuts, 1 tablespoon honey. Serve and enjoy!

NUTRITION: Calories: 295 Fat: 8g Carbohydrates: 56g Protein: 6g

6. Tomato and Dill Frittata

Preparation time: 5 minutes

Cooking time: 10 minutes

Servings: 4

INGREDIENTS:

- 2 tablespoons olive oil
- 1 medium onion, chopped
- 1 teaspoon garlic, minced
- 2 medium tomatoes, chopped
- 6 large eggs
- ½ cup half and half
- ½ cup feta cheese, crumbled
- ¼ cup dill weed
- Salt as needed
- Ground black pepper as needed

DIRECTIONS:

1. Pre-heat your oven to a temperature of 400 degrees Fahrenheit. Take a large sized ovenproof pan and heat up your olive oil over medium-high heat. Toss in the onion, garlic, tomatoes and stir fry them for 4 minutes.

2. While they are being cooked, take a bowl and beat together your eggs, half and half cream and season the mix with some pepper and salt.

3. Pour the mixture into the pan with your vegetables and top it with crumbled feta cheese and dill weed. Cover it with the lid and let it cook for 3 minutes.

4. Place the pan inside your oven and let it bake for 10 minutes. Serve hot.

NUTRITION: Calories: 191 Fat: 15g Carbohydrates: 6g Protein: 9g

7. Strawberry and Rhubarb Smoothie

Preparation time: 5 minutes

Cooking time: 3 minutes

Servings: 1

INGREDIENTS:

- 1 rhubarb stalk, chopped
- 1 cup fresh strawberries, sliced
- ½ cup plain Greek strawberries
- Pinch of ground cinnamon
- 3 ice cubes

DIRECTIONS:

1. Take a small saucepan and fill with water over high heat. Bring to boil and add rhubarb, boil for 3 minutes. Drain and transfer to blender.
2. Add strawberries, honey, yogurt, cinnamon and pulse mixture until smooth. Add ice cubes and blend until thick with no lumps. Pour into glass and enjoy chilled.

NUTRITION: Calories: 295 Fat: 8g Carbohydrates: 56g Protein: 6g

8. Bacon and Brie Omelet Wedges

Preparation time: 10 minutes

Cooking time: 10 minutes

Servings: 6

INGREDIENTS:

- 2 tablespoons olive oil

- 7 ounces smoked bacon

- 6 beaten eggs

- Small bunch chives, snipped

- 3 ½ ounces brie, sliced

- 1 teaspoon red wine vinegar

- 1 teaspoon Dijon mustard

- 1 cucumber, halved, deseeded and sliced diagonally

- 7 ounces radish, quartered

DIRECTIONS:

1. Turn your grill on and set it to high. Take a small-sized pan and add 1 teaspoon of oil, allow the oil to heat up. Add lardons and fry until crisp. Drain the lardon on kitchen paper.

2. Take another non-sticky cast iron frying pan and place it over grill, heat 2 teaspoons of oil. Add lardons, eggs, chives, ground pepper to the frying pan. Cook on low until they are semi-set.

3. Carefully lay brie on top and grill until the Brie sets and is a golden texture. Remove it from the pan and cut up into wedges.

4. Take a small bowl and create dressing by mixing olive oil, mustard, vinegar and seasoning. Add cucumber to the bowl and mix, serve alongside the omelet wedges.

NUTRITION: Calories: 35 Fat: 31g Carbohydrates: 3g Protein: 25g

9. Pearl Couscous Salad

Preparation time: 15 minutes

Cooking time: 0 minutes

Servings: 6

INGREDIENTS:

- For Lemon Dill Vinaigrette:
- Juice of 1 large sized lemon
- 1/3 cup of extra virgin olive oil
- 1 teaspoon of dill weed
- 1 teaspoon of garlic powder
- Salt as needed
- Pepper
- For Israeli Couscous:
- 2 cups of Pearl Couscous
- Extra virgin olive oil
- 2 cups of halved grape tomatoes
- Water as needed
- 1/3 cup of finely chopped red onions
- ½ of a finely chopped English cucumber
- 15 ounces of chickpeas
- 14 ounce can of artichoke hearts (roughly chopped up)
- ½ cup of pitted Kalamata olives
- 15-20 pieces of fresh basil leaves, roughly torn and chopped up
- 3 ounces of fresh baby mozzarella

DIRECTIONS:

1. Prepare the vinaigrette by taking a bowl and add the ingredients listed under vinaigrette. Mix them well and keep aside. Take a medium-sized heavy pot and place it over medium heat.

2. Add 2 tablespoons of olive oil and allow it to heat up. Add couscous and keep cooking until golden brown. Add 3 cups of boiling water and cook the couscous according to the package instructions.

3. Once done, drain in a colander and keep aside. Take another large-sized mixing bowl and add the remaining ingredients except the cheese and basil.

4. Add the cooked couscous and basil to the mix and mix everything well. Give the vinaigrette a nice stir and whisk it into the couscous salad. Mix well.

5. Adjust the seasoning as required. Add mozzarella cheese. Garnish with some basil. Enjoy!

NUTRITION: Calories: 393 Fat: 13g Carbohydrates: 57g Protein: 13g

10. Coconut Porridge

Preparation time: 15 minutes

Cooking time: 0 minutes

Servings: 6

INGREDIENTS:

- Powdered erythritol as needed
- 1 ½ cups almond milk, unsweetened
- 2 tablespoons vanilla protein powder
- 3 tablespoons Golden Flaxseed meal
- 2 tablespoons coconut flour

DIRECTIONS:

1. Take a bowl and mix in flaxseed meal, protein powder, coconut flour and mix well. Add mix to saucepan (placed over medium heat).

2. Add almond milk and stir, let the mixture thicken. Add your desired amount of sweetener and serve. Enjoy!

NUTRITION: Calories: 259 Fat: 13g Carbohydrates: 5g Protein: 16g

11. Crumbled Feta and Scallions

Preparation time: 5 minutes

Cooking time: 15 minutes

Servings: 12

INGREDIENTS:

- 2 tablespoons of unsalted butter (replace with canola oil for full effect)
- ½ cup of chopped up scallions
- 1 cup of crumbled feta cheese
- 8 large sized eggs
- 2/3 cup of milk
- ½ teaspoon of dried Italian seasoning
- Salt as needed
- Freshly ground black pepper as needed
- Cooking oil spray

DIRECTIONS:

1. Pre-heat your oven to 400 degrees Fahrenheit. Take a 3-4 ounce muffin pan and grease with cooking oil. Take a non-stick pan and place it over medium heat.

2. Add butter and allow the butter to melt. Add half of the scallions and stir fry. Keep them to the side. Take a medium-sized bowl and add eggs, Italian seasoning and milk and whisk well.

3. Add the stir fried scallions and feta cheese and mix. Season with pepper and salt. Pour the mix into the muffin tin. Transfer the muffin tin to your oven and bake for 15 minutes. Serve with a sprinkle of scallions.

NUTRITION: Calories: 106 Fat: 8g Carbohydrates: 2g Protein: 7g

12. Quinoa Chicken Salad

Preparation time: 15 minutes

Cooking time: 20 minutes

Servings: 8

INGREDIENTS:

- 2 cups of water
- 2 cubes of chicken bouillon
- 1 smashed garlic clove
- 1 cup of uncooked quinoa
- 2 large sized chicken breasts cut up into bite-sized portions and cooked
- 1 large sized diced red onion

- 1 large sized green bell pepper
- ½ cup of Kalamata olives
- ½ cup of crumbled feta cheese
- ¼ cup of chopped up parsley
- ¼ cup of chopped up fresh chives
- ½ teaspoon of salt
- 1 tablespoon of balsamic vinegar
- ¼ cup of olive oil

DIRECTIONS:

1. Take a saucepan and bring your water, garlic and bouillon cubes to a boil. Stir in quinoa and reduce the heat to medium low.
2. Simmer for about 15-20 minutes until the quinoa has absorbed all the water and is tender. Discard your garlic cloves and scrape the quinoa into a large sized bowl.
3. Gently stir in the cooked chicken breast, bell pepper, onion, feta cheese, chives, salt and parsley into your quinoa.
4. Drizzle some lemon juice, olive oil and balsamic vinegar. Stir everything until mixed well. Serve warm and enjoy!

NUTRITION: Calories: 99 Fat: 7g Carbohydrates: 7g Protein: 3.4g

13. Gnocchi Ham Olives

Preparation time: 5 minutes

Cooking time: 15 minutes

Servings: 4

INGREDIENTS:

- 2 tablespoons of olive oil
- 1 medium-sized onion chopped up
- 3 minced cloves of garlic
- 1 medium-sized red pepper completely deseeded and finely chopped
- 1 cup of tomato puree
- 2 tablespoons of tomato paste
- 1 pound of gnocchi
- 1 cup of coarsely chopped turkey ham
- ½ cup of sliced pitted olives
- 1 teaspoon of Italian seasoning
- Salt as needed
- Freshly ground black pepper
- Bunch of fresh basil leaves

DIRECTIONS:

1. Take a medium-sized sauce pan and place over medium-high heat. Pour some olive oil and heat it up. Toss in the bell pepper, onion and garlic and sauté for 2 minutes.

2. Pour in the tomato puree, gnocchi, tomato paste and add the turkey ham, Italian seasoning and olives. Simmer the whole mix for 15 minutes, making sure to stir from time to time.

3. Season the mix with some pepper and salt. Once done, transfer the mix to a dish and garnish with some basil leaves. Serve hot and have fun.

NUTRITION: Calories: 335 Fat: 12g Carbohydrates: 45g Protein: 15g

14. Spicy Early Morning Seafood Risotto

Preparation time: 5 minutes

Cooking time: 15 minutes

Servings: 4

INGREDIENTS:

- 3 cups of clam juice
- 2 cups of water
- 2 tablespoons of olive oil
- 1 medium-sized chopped up onion
- 2 minced cloves of garlic
- 1 ½ cups of Arborio Rice
- ½ cup of dry white wine
- 1 teaspoon of Saffron
- ½ teaspoon of ground cumin
- ½ teaspoon of paprika
- 1 pound of marinara seafood mix
- Salt as needed
- Ground pepper as needed

DIRECTIONS:

1. Place a saucepan over high heat and pour in your clam juice with water and bring the mixture to a boil. Remove the heat.
2. Take a heavy bottomed saucepan and stir fry your garlic and onion in oil over medium heat until a nice fragrance comes off.

3. Add in the rice and keep stirring for 2-3 minutes until the rice has been fully covered with the oil. Pour the wine and then add the saffron.

4. Keep stirring constantly until it is fully absorbed. Add in the cumin, clam juice, paprika mixture 1 cup at a time, making sure to keep stirring it from time to time.

5. Cook the rice for 20 minutes until perfect. Finally, add the seafood marinara mix and cook for another 5-7 minutes.

6. Season with some pepper and salt. Transfer the meal to a serving dish. Serve hot.

NUTRITION: Calories: 386 Fat: 7g Carbohydrates: 55g Protein: 21g

15. Rocket Tomatoes and Mushroom Frittata

Preparation time: 5 minutes

Cooking time: 15 minutes

Servings: 4

INGREDIENTS:

- 2 tablespoons of butter (replace with canola oil for full effect)
- 1 chopped up medium-sized onion
- 2 minced cloves of garlic
- 1 cup of coarsely chopped baby rocket tomato
- 1 cup of sliced button mushrooms
- 6 large pieces of eggs
- ½ cup of skim milk

- 1 teaspoon of dried rosemary
- Salt as needed
- Ground black pepper as needed

DIRECTIONS:

1. Pre-heat your oven to 400 degrees Fahrenheit. Take a large oven-proof pan and place it over medium-heat. Heat up some oil.

2. Stir fry your garlic, onion for about 2 minutes. Add the mushroom, rosemary and rockets and cook for 3 minutes. Take a medium-sized bowl and beat your eggs alongside the milk.

3. Season it with some salt and pepper. Pour the egg mixture into your pan with the vegetables and sprinkle some Parmesan.

4. Reduce the heat to low and cover with the lid. Let it cook for 3 minutes. Transfer the pan into your oven and bake for 10 minutes until fully settled.

5. Reduce the heat to low and cover with your lid. Let it cook for 3 minutes. Transfer the pan into your oven and then bake for another 10 minutes. Serve hot.

NUTRITION: Calories: 189 Fat: 13g Carbohydrates: 6g Protein: 12g

APPETIZER AND SNACK

RECIPES

16. Thin-Crust Flatbread

Preparation time: 15 minutes

Cooking time: 25 minutes

Servings: 2

INGREDIENTS:

- 2 cup all-purpose flour
- ¾ cup lukewarm water
- 1 teaspoon instant yeast
- 1 ½ teaspoon salt
- 1 tablespoon olive oil
- 1 garlic clove, crushed
- ¼ teaspoon sea salt
- ½ tomato, thinly sliced
- ¼ yellow beet, thinly sliced
- ½ Meyer lemon, thinly sliced
- ¼ potato, thinly sliced
- 1 radish, thinly sliced
- ½ burrata mozzarella ball, dotted all over flatbread

- 1 tablespoon fresh tarragon, chopped

DIRECTIONS:

1. Mix yeast and water in a bowl and stir to dissolve the yeast. Add salt and flour to the bowl and mix well.

2. Turn the dough onto a clear surface. Knead well for 5 minutes. If dough is sticky, add 1 tablespoon flour at a time. Let the dough rise for 1 ½ hour. Cover with a bowl. Preheat the oven to 375F.

3. Roll out the flatbread. Brush olive oil over it. Rub crushed garlic over it. Sprinkle with sea salt. Lay toppings over it as you like.

4. Dollop cheese over it. Sprinkle with pinches of salt. Place in the oven and bake for 25 minutes. Top with tarragon. Serve.

NUTRITION: Calories: 150 Carbs: 27g Fat: 2g Protein: 7g

17. Smoked Salmon Goat Cheese Endive Bites

Preparation time: 15 minutes

Cooking time: 0 minutes

Servings: 4

INGREDIENTS:

- 1 package herbed goat cheese
- 3 endive heads
- 1 package smoked salmon

DIRECTIONS:

1. Pull the leaves apart from endives and cut the ends off of them. Add goat cheese to endive leaves. Add salmon slices on top of the goat cheese.Serve.

NUTRITION: Calories: 46 Carbs: 1g Fat: 3g Protein: 3g

18. Hummus Peppers

Preparation time: 15 minutes

Cooking time: 0 minutes

Servings: 12

INGREDIENTS:

- 6 baby bell peppers, halved lengthwise
- 10 oz. hummus
- ¼ cup kalamata olives, pitted and chopped
- ¼ cup reduced fat crumbled feta
- parsley

DIRECTIONS:

1. Place sliced bell peppers in a plate and add 2 tablespoons of hummus to each. Add feta, olives and parsley. Serve.

NUTRITION: Calories: 70 Carbs: 4g Fat: 5g Protein: 2g

19. Loaded Mediterranean Hummus

Preparation time: 15 minutes

Cooking time: 0 minutes

Servings: 2 cups

INGREDIENTS:

- 1 tablespoon olive oil
- 2 cups hummus
- 1 teaspoon paprika
- 1 cup olives, sliced
- ½ red bell pepper, sliced
- 2 tablespoon pine nuts
- 2 tablespoon cilantros, chopped
- ¼ cup feta cheese, crumbled

DIRECTIONS:

1. Add hummus to a serving dish. Add paprika and olive oil. Add olives, red bell pepper, feta cheese, pine nuts and cilantro, then mix well. Serve.

NUTRITION: Calories: 70 Carbs: 4g Fat: 5g Protein: 2g

20. Smoky Loaded Eggplant Dip

Preparation time: 15 minutes

Cooking time: 20 minutes

Servings: 6

INGREDIENTS:

- 1 large eggplant
- 1 ½ tablespoon Greek yoghurt
- 2 tablespoon tahini paste
- 1 garlic clove, chopped
- 1 tablespoon lemon juice
- 1 ½ teaspoon sumac

- ¾ teaspoon Aleppo pepper
- toasted pine nuts
- salt and pepper
- 1 tomato, diced
- ½ English cucumber, diced
- lemon juice
- parsley
- olive oil

DIRECTIONS:

1. Add parsley, cucumber and tomato to a bowl. Season with ½ teaspoon sumac, salt and pepper. Add lemon juice and olive oil. Toss and set aside.

2. Turn a gas burner on high and turn eggplant on it every 5 minutes with a tong until charred and crispy, for 20 minutes. Remove from the heat and let cool.

3. Peel the skin off the eggplant and discard the stem. Transfer eggplant flesh to a colander and drain for 5 minutes.

4. Transfer flesh to a blender. Add yoghurt, tahini paste, garlic, lemon juice, salt, pepper, Aleppo pepper and sumac. Blend for 2 pulses to combine.

5. Transfer to a bowl. Cover and refrigerate for 30 minutes. Bring it to a room temperature and add olive oil on top. Add pine nuts. Add salad on top and serve.

NUTRITION: Calories: 40 Carbs: 3g Fat: 4g Protein: 0g

21. Peanut Butter Banana Greek Yogurt Bowl

Preparation time: 15 minutes

Cooking time: 0 minutes

Servings: 4

INGREDIENTS:

- 2 medium bananas, sliced
- 4 cups vanilla Greek yoghurt
- ¼ cup peanut butter
- 1 teaspoon nutmeg
- ¼ cup flax seed meal

DIRECTIONS:

1. Divide the yoghurt equally among 4 bowls and add banana slices to it. Add peanut butter to a bowl and microwave for 40 seconds.
2. Add 1 tablespoon peanut butter over each bowl. Add nutmeg and flax seed meal to each bowl. Serve.

NUTRITION: Calories: 110 Carbs: 13g Fat: 0g Protein: 15g

22. Roasted Chickpeas

Preparation time: 15 minutes

Cooking time: 30 minutes

Servings: 2

INGREDIENTS:

- 2 tablespoons extra virgin olive oil

- 2 15 oz. cans chickpeas

- 2 teaspoon red wine vinegar

- 2 teaspoon lemon juice

- 1 teaspoon dried oregano

- ½ teaspoon garlic powder

- 1 teaspoon kosher salt

- ½ teaspoon black pepper, cracked

DIRECTIONS:

1. Preheat the oven to 425F and line a baking sheet with parchment paper. Drain, rinse and dry chickpeas and put on a baking sheet.

2. Roast for 10 minutes, then remove from the oven. Turn chickpeas and roast for 10 minutes. Add the remaining ingredients to a bowl and mix well.

3. Add chickpeas to it and mix to coat well. Transfer coated chickpeas back to the oven and roast for 10 minutes. Cool completely. Serve.

NUTRITION: Calories: 191 Carbs: 27g Fat: 1g Protein: 9g

23. Savory Feta Spinach and Sweet Red Pepper Muffins

Preparation time: 15 minutes

Cooking time: 25 minutes

Servings: 12

INGREDIENTS:

- 2 eggs
- 2 ¾ cups all-purpose flour
- ¼ cup sugar
- 1 teaspoon paprika
- 2 teaspoons baking powder
- ¾ cup low-fat milk
- ½ cup extra virgin olive oil
- ¾ cup feta, crumbled
- 1/3 cup jarred florina peppers, drained and patted dry
- ¾ teaspoon salt
- 1 ¼ cup spinach, thinly sliced

DIRECTIONS:

1. Preheat the oven to 375F. Mix sugar, flour, baking powder, paprika and salt in a bowl. Mix eggs, olive oil and milk in another bowl.

2. Add wet ingredients to dry and mix until blended. Add spinach, feta and peppers and mix well.

3. Line a muffin pan with liners and add the mixture to them equally. Bake for 25 minutes. Let cool for 10 minutes. Remove from the tray. Cool for 2 hours and serve.

NUTRITION: Calories: 295 Carbs: 27g Fat: 18g Protein: 8g

24. Baked Whole-Grain Lavash Chips with Dip

Preparation time: 15 minutes

Cooking time: 6 minutes

Servings: 4

INGREDIENTS:

- 3 teaspoon oil
- 3 California lavash whole-grain lavash flatbreads, cut into 16 squares
- 1 ripe avocado
- ½ cup cashews, soaked overnight, drained and rinsed
- ½ cup parsley, chopped
- 2 garlic cloves
- ½ cup kalamata olive brine
- ¼ cup tahini
- 1 lemon juice
- salt and pepper
- cherry tomatoes

DIRECTIONS:

1. Blend cashews, avocado, garlic and parsley in a blender. Add lemon juice, olive brine, tahini and blend well. Season. Transfer to a bowl and add parsley. Set aside.

2. Preheat the oven to 400F and place lavash squares on top. Add little oil on both sides of each squares. Bake for 6 minutes and remove from the oven Let cool.

3. Chop cherry tomatoes. Serve chips with tomatoes and dip.

NUTRITION: Calories: 557 Carbs: 33g Fat: 30g Protein: 35g

25. Quinoa Granola

Preparation time: 15 minutes

Cooking time: 35 minutes

Servings: 7

INGREDIENTS:

- 1 cup old fashioned rolled oats
- 2 cups raw almonds, chopped
- ½ cup white quinoa, uncooked
- 1 tablespoon coconut sugar
- 3 ½ tablespoon coconut oil
- ¼ cup maple syrup
- pinch sea salt

DIRECTIONS:

1. Preheat the oven to 340F. Add quinoa, oats, almonds, sugar and salt to a bowl. Mix well. Add maple syrup and coconut oil to a pan. Heat over medium heat for 3 minutes, whisking along.

2. Add dry ingredients and stir to coat well. Place on a baking sheet and spread. Bake for 20 minutes. Remove from the oven and toss the granola.

3. Turn pan around and bake for 8 minutes more. Cool completely and serve.

NUTRITION: Calories: 274 Carbs: 38g Fat: 11g Protein: 9g

26. Greek Yogurt Spinach Artichoke Dip

Preparation time: 15 minutes

Cooking time: 30 minutes

Servings: 16

INGREDIENTS:

- 10 0z. package frozen spinach, thawed
- 1 1/3 cups plain Greek yoghurt
- 14 oz. can artichoke hearts, drained and chopped
- 2 garlic cloves, minced
- 6 oz. feta, crumbled
- 1/3 cup parmesan, shredded
- 2/3 cup mozzarella, shredded

DIRECTIONS:

1. Preheat the oven to 350F and grease a 1 quart casserole dish. Set aside. Drain out the liquid from spinach completely. Add spinach to a bowl.
2. Add the remaining ingredients and mix well. Transfer the mixture to a baking dish. Add more parmesan and mozzarella. Bake for 30 minutes. Serve.

NUTRITION: Calories: 50 Carbs: 2g Fat: 5g Protein: 2g

27. Fig Smoothie with Cinnamon

Preparation time: 5 minutes

Cooking time: 0 minutes

Servings: 1

INGREDIENTS:

- 1 large ripe fig
- 3 dessertspoons porridge oats
- 3 rounded dessertspoons Greek yoghurt
- ½ teaspoon ground cinnamon
- 200 ml orange juice
- 3 ice cubes

DIRECTIONS:

1. Wash and dry the fig. Chop. Add all ingredients to a blender. Blend well. Serve.

NUTRITION: Calories: 152 Carbs: 32g Fat: 3g Protein: 3g

28. Smoked Salmon, Avocado and Cucumber Bites

Preparation time: 15 minutes

Cooking time: 0 minutes

Servings: 12

INGREDIENTS:

- 1 large avocado, peeled and pit removed
- 1 medium cucumber

- ½ tablespoon lime juice

- 6 oz. smoked salmon

- chives

- black pepper

DIRECTIONS:

1. Cut cucumber into ¼ inch thick slices. Place flat on a plate. Add lime juice, avocado to a bowl and mash well.

2. Spread avocado on each cucumber slice and add a slice of smoked salmon on top. Add chives and black pepper on top. Serve.

NUTRITION: Calories: 216 Carbs: 6g Fat: 10g Protein: 27g

29. Baked Root Vegetable Chips with Buttermilk-Parsley Dipping Sauce

Preparation time: 15 minutes

Cooking time: 40 minutes

Servings: 2

INGREDIENTS:

- 6 tablespoons buttermilk

- 7 oz. cup 2% Greek yoghurt

- 2 tablespoons parsley, minced

- 2 garlic cloves, minced

- 1 teaspoon honey

- 1 teaspoon lemon zest

- salt

- 1 large parsnip
- 1 medium turnip
- 1 medium golden beet
- 1 medium red beet
- 2 tablespoons olive oil
- 1 teaspoon garlic powder
- ½ teaspoon dried thyme
- ½ teaspoon ground cumin
- ¼ teaspoon kosher salt

DIRECTIONS:

1. Whisk first 7 ingredients in a bowl and mix until combined. Cover and refrigerate. Preheat the oven to 400F. Mix dried thyme, oil, garlic powder, ground cumin and kosher salt in a bowl.

2. Peel all of the root vegetables and slice them 1/8 inch thick.Brush oil on both sides of chips, place slices on a wire rack and place the wire rack on 2 baking sheets.

3. Place baking sheets in oven and bake until crispy. Check on them every 20 minutes and remove once done. Serve with sauce.

NUTRITION: Calories: 506 Carbs: 67g Fat: 26g Protein: 3g

30. Spicy Red Lentil Dip

Preparation time: 15 minutes

Cooking time: 20 minutes

Servings: 6

INGREDIENTS:

- 1 cup red lentils, picked over and rinsed
- 1 teaspoon onion powder
- 2 teaspoons curry powder
- ¼ teaspoon turmeric
- ½ teaspoon cumin
- ½ teaspoon garam masala
- 1 teaspoon sea salt
- ¼ teaspoon black pepper
- crackers

DIRECTIONS:

1. Add red lentils to a pan and cover with water by one inch.Bring to a boil and reduce the heat to medium low. Cook for 20 minutes. Mash lentils.
2. Add all spices and mix well. Serve with crackers.

NUTRITION: Calories: 79 Carbs: 0g Fat: 5g Protein: 3g

31. Cucumber Hummus Sandwiches

Preparation time: 15 minutes

Cooking time: 0 minutes

Servings: 1

INGREDIENTS:

- 10 round slices English cucumber
- 5 teaspoons hummus

DIRECTIONS:

1. Add 1 teaspoon hummus to a slice of cucumber and top with another cucumber. Repeat with the rest. Serve.

NUTRITION: Calories: 108 Carbs: 13g Fat: 5g Protein: 3g

32. Fig & Honey Yogurt

Preparation time: 15 minutes

Cooking time: 0 minutes

Servings: 1

INGREDIENTS:

- 3 dried figs, sliced
- 2 teaspoons honey
- 2/3 cup low-fat plain yoghurt

DIRECTIONS:

1. Add yoghurt to a bowl and top with honey and figs. Serve.

NUTRITION: Calories: 240 Carbs: 29g Fat: 9g Protein: 7g

33. Peach Caprese Skewers

Preparation time: 15 minutes

Cooking time: 0 minutes

Servings: 1

INGREDIENTS:

- ½ cup cherry tomatoes
- 1 medium peach, sliced
- ¼ cup baby mozzarella balls
- 4 fresh basil leaves

DIRECTIONS:

1. Put peach slices, tomatoes, basil and mozzarella balls on skewers. Serve.

NUTRITION: Calories: 103 Carbs: 10g Fat: 4g Protein: 7g

34. Tomato-Basil Skewers

Preparation time: 15 minutes

Cooking time: 0 minutes

Servings: 16

INGREDIENTS:

- 16 cherry tomatoes
- 16 small mozzarella balls
- 16 fresh basil leaves
- extra virgin olive oil
- salt and black pepper

DIRECTIONS:

1. Put basil, tomatoes and mozzarella balls on skewers. Add oil and season with salt and pepper. Serve.

NUTRITION: Calories: 106 Carbs: 3g Fat: 7g Protein: 7g

35. Fig & Ricotta Toast

Preparation time: 15 minutes

Cooking time: 5 minutes

Servings: 1

INGREDIENTS:

- 1 slice whole-grain bread, 1/2 "thick
- 1 teaspoon honey
- ¼ cup part-skim ricotta cheese
- 1 teaspoon sliced almonds, roasted
- 1 fresh fig
- pinch of sea salt

DIRECTIONS:

1. Toast bread. Add cheese, figs and almonds on top. Add honey and season with salt. Serve.

NUTRITION: Calories: 240 Carbs: 36g Fat: 8g Protein: 8g

MAIN RECIPES: SEAFOOD

36. Pasta with Cherry Tomatoes and Anchovies

Preparation time: 15 minutes

Cooking time: 20 minutes

Servings: 5

INGREDIENTS:

- 10 ½ oz Spaghetti
- 1 1/8-pound Cherry tomatoes
- 9oz Anchovies (pre-cleaned)
- 2 tablespoons Capers
- 1 clove of garlic
- 1 Small red onion
- Parsley to taste
- Extra virgin olive oil to taste
- Table salt to taste
- Black pepper to taste
- Black olives to taste

DIRECTIONS:

1. Cut the garlic clove, obtaining thin slices. Cut the cherry tomatoes in 2. Peel the onion and slice it thinly.

2. Put a little oil with the sliced garlic and onions in a saucepan. Heat everything over medium heat for 5 minutes; stir occasionally.

3. Once everything has been well flavored, add the cherry tomatoes and a pinch of salt and pepper. Cook for 15 minutes.

4. Meanwhile, put a pot of water on the stove and as soon as it boils, add the salt and the pasta. Once the sauce is almost ready, add the anchovies and cook for a couple of minutes. Stir gently.

5. Turn off the heat, chop the parsley and place it in the pan. When the pasta is cooked, strain it and add it directly to the sauce. Turn the heat back on again for a few seconds. Serve.

NUTRITION: Calories 446 Carbs 66.1g Protein 22.8g Fat 10g

37. <u>Mussels with Tomatoes & Chili</u>

Preparation time: 15 minutes

Cooking time: 12 minutes

Servings: 4

INGREDIENTS:

- 2 ripe tomatoes
- 2 tbsps. olive oil
- 1 tsp. tomato paste
- 1 garlic clove, chopped
- 1 shallot, chopped
- 1 chopped red or green chili
- A small glass of dry white wine

- Salt and pepper to taste
- 2 lbs./900 g. mussels, cleaned
- Basil leaves, fresh

DIRECTIONS:

1. Add tomatoes to boiling water for 3 minutes then drain. Peel the tomatoes and chop the flesh. Add oil to an iron skillet and heat to sauté shallots and garlic for 3 minutes.

2. Stir in wine along with tomatoes, chili, salt/pepper and tomato paste. Cook for 2 minutes then add mussels. Cover and let it steam for 4 minutes. Garnish with basil leaves and serve warm.

NUTRITION: Calories 483 Fat 15.2 g Carbs 20.4 g Protein 62.3 g

38. Lemon Garlic Shrimp

Preparation time: 15 minutes

Cooking time: 10 minutes

Servings: 6

INGREDIENTS:

- 4 tsps. extra-virgin olive oil, divided
- 2 red bell peppers, diced
- 2 lbs./900 g. fresh asparagus, sliced
- 2 tsps. lemon zest, freshly grated
- ½ tsp. salt, divided
- 5 garlic cloves, minced
- 1 lb./450 g. peeled raw shrimp, deveined
- 1 c. reduced-sodium chicken broth or water

- 1 tsp. cornstarch
- 2 tbsps. lemon juice
- 2 tbsps. fresh parsley, chopped

DIRECTIONS:

1. Add 2 teaspoon oil to a large skillet and heat for a minute. Stir in asparagus, lemon zest, bell pepper and salt. Sauté for 6 minutes.
2. Keep the sautéed veggies in a separate bowl. Add remaining oil in the same pan and add garlic.Sauté for 30 seconds then add shrimp. Cook for 1 minute.
3. Mix cornstarch with broth in a bowl and pour this mixture into the pan. Add salt and stir cook for 2 minutes. Turn off flame then add parsley and lemon juice. Serve warm with sautéed vegetables.

NUTRITION: Calories 204 Fat 4 g Carbs 23.6 g Protein 17. 1 g

39. Pepper Tilapia with Spinach

Preparation time: 15 minutes

Cooking time: 27 minutes

Servings: 4

INGREDIENTS:

- 4 tilapia fillets, 8 oz./ 227 g. each
- 4 cups fresh spinach
- 1 red onion, sliced
- 3 garlic cloves, minced
- 2 tbsps. extra virgin olive oil

- 3 lemons
- 1 tbsp. ground black pepper
- 1 tbsp. ground white pepper
- 1 tbsp. crushed red pepper

DIRECTIONS:

1. Set the oven to preheat at 350°F/176.6°C. Place the fish in a shallow baking dish and juice two of the lemons.

2. Cover the fish in the lemon juice and then sprinkle the three types of pepper over the fish. Slice the remaining lemon and cover the fish. Bake in the oven for 20 minutes.

3. While the fish cooks, sauté the garlic and onion in the olive oil. Add the spinach and sauté for 7 more minutes. Top the fish with spinach and serve.

NUTRITION: Calories 323 Fat 11.4 g Carbs 10.4 g Protein 50 g

40. Spicy Shrimp Salad

Preparation time: 15 minutes

Cooking time: 0 minutes

Servings: 2

INGREDIENTS:

- ½ lb. salad shrimp, chopped
- 2 stalks celery, chopped
- ¼ cup red onion, diced
- 1 tsp. black pepper
- 1 tsp. red pepper

- 1 tbsp. lemon juice
- Dash of cayenne pepper
- 1 tbsp. olive oil
- 2 cucumbers, sliced

DIRECTIONS:

1. Combine the shrimp, celery, and onion in a bowl and mix together. In a separate bowl, whisk the oil and the lemon juice, then add red pepper, black pepper, and cayenne pepper.
2. Pour over the shrimp and mix. Serve with slices of thickly cut cucumber on it and enjoy.

NUTRITION: Calories: 245 Fat: 9g Carbs: 18.2g Protein: 27.3g

41. Baked Cod in Parchment

Preparation time: 15 minutes

Cooking time: 0 minutes

Servings: 1

INGREDIENTS:

- 1-2 potatoes, sliced
- 5 cherry tomatoes, halved
- 5 pitted olives
- Juice of ½ lemon
- ½ tbsp. olive oil
- 4 oz. cod
- 20 inches long parchment
- Sea salt and black pepper

DIRECTIONS:

1. Set your oven to preheat at 350°F/176.6°C. Spread the olive oil on parchment and arrange potato on it.

2. In separate bowl combine the tomatoes, olives, and lemon juice. Put the fish fillet on potatoes and top with tomato mixture. Add salt and pepper. Fold the filled parchment squares and bake for 20 minutes.

NUTRITION: Calories 330 Fat 8 g Carbs 35 g Protein 25 g

42. Thai Tuna Bowl

Preparation time: 15 minutes

Cooking time: 0 minutes

Servings: 1

INGREDIENTS:

- ½ cup cooked quinoa, at room temperature
- ½ cup spiralized zucchini
- 1 carrot, spiralized
- ¼ cup chopped red cabbage
- 2 tbsps. diced red onion
- ¼ cup roasted chickpeas
- 5 1/2 oz White Albacore Tuna, drained
- Cilantro
- Juice of 1 lime
- Simple Thai Peanut Dressing

DIRECTIONS:

1. Add quinoa to the bottom of a large bowl. Add zucchini noodles, cabbage, onion, chickpeas, tuna, and carrot to the bowl. Top with cilantro and lime juice. Stir in a peanut dressing and serve.

NUTRITION: Calories 246 Fat 7.4 g Carbs 15.3 g Protein 12.4g

43. Roasted Fish & New Potatoes

Preparation time: 15 minutes

Cooking time: 35 minutes

Servings: 4

INGREDIENTS:

- 3 tbsps. extra-virgin olive oil
- 3 tbsps. orange juice
- 3 tbsps. white vinegar
- ½ tsp. orange peel, grated
- ¼ tsp. dried dillweed
- 12 new potatoes, cubed
- 4 salmon fillets, skin removed

DIRECTIONS:

1. Preheat oven to 420°F/215°C. Blend first five ingredients. Sprinkle potato with 2 tbsps. of this mixture. Bake for 20 minutes.
2. Sprinkle fillets with remaining mixture and add to the potatoes. Cook for about 15 minutes and serve.

NUTRITION: Calories 289 Fat 8.2 g Carbs 23.4 g Protein 29 g

44. Pecan-Crusted Catfish

Preparation time: 15 minutes

Cooking time: 10 minutes

Servings: 4

INGREDIENTS:

- 2 medium eggs
- 2 tbsps. water
- 4 catfish fillets
- ½ cup flour
- 1 cup pecans, chopped
- 2 tbsps. extra-virgin olive oil
- Salt and pepper

DIRECTIONS:

1. Combine egg and water. Put fish in the mixture and let sit while preparing other ingredients. Put flour on one sheet of wax paper, pecans on another.

2. Take each fish fillet from the egg mixture. Coat one side of fish in flour, other in pecans. Cook fillets in the skillet for 5 minutes on each side.

NUTRITION: Calories 355 Fat 19.3 g Carbs 14.1 g Protein 30.7 g

45. Skillet Shrimp

Preparation time: 15 minutes

Cooking time: 10 minutes

Servings: 4

INGREDIENTS:

- 1 lb. peeled shrimp, deveined
- 2 tbsps. extra-virgin olive oil
- 2 cloves garlic, chopped
- 1 tsp. dried thyme
- 1 onion, sliced
- Salt and pepper

DIRECTIONS:

1. Set olive oil, onion and garlic in a skillet. Heat for 3 minutes. Stir in the shrimp, thyme, salt, and pepper.
2. Cook for 6 minutes in the pan under the broiler (8 inches from the heat source).

NUTRITION: Calories 200 Carbs 5g Fat 9g Protein 24g

46. Shrimp & Feta

Preparation time: 15 minutes

Cooking time: 0 minutes

Servings: 4

INGREDIENTS:

- 1 onion, sliced
- 1 green pepper, sliced
- 2 cloves garlic, chopped
- 4 tbsps. olive oil
- 2 tomatoes, cubed
- 1 lb. deveined shrimp, peeled

- 8 oz. cubed feta
- Salt and pepper

DIRECTIONS:

1. Sauté the green pepper, garlic, and onion in olive oil for 5 minutes. Stir in tomatoes and simmer for 15 minutes. Add shrimp and feta. Season with salt and pepper to taste. Cook for another 15 minutes.

NUTRITION: Calories 320 Fat 20 g Carbs 10 g Protein 26 g

47. White Fish with Herbs

Preparation time: 15 minutes

Cooking time: 5 minutes

Servings: 4

INGREDIENTS:

- 2 tbsps. olive oil
- 2 tbsps. butter
- 4 fresh fish fillets
- Juice of 2 large lemons
- 3 tbsps. capers
- ½ cup chopped fresh parsley, mint (or any other fresh herbs you prefer)
- Salt and pepper to taste

DIRECTIONS:

1. Set heat to medium-high. Set a non-stick pan in place and add the olive oil and butter, allow the butter to melt and become slightly frothy.

2. Add in the fish and fry on both sides for about 2 minutes or until golden and almost cooked through.

3. Add the lemon juice and capers, and allow the acid of the lemon juice to deglaze the pan. Add the fresh herbs, salt and pepper just before you remove the pan from the heat and serve.

4. Serve with a little extra butter and a wedge of lemon.

NUTRITION: Calories 282 Fat 15 g Carbs 2.6 g Protein 35.2 g

48. <u>Grilled White Fish with Fresh Basil Pesto</u>

Preparation time: 15 minutes

Cooking time: 15 minutes

Servings: 4

INGREDIENTS:

- 1 cup fresh basil leaves
- 4 tbsps. olive oil
- ¼ cup grated parmesan
- ¼ cup toasted pine nuts
- Juice of ½ lemon
- Salt & pepper
- 4 fresh white fish fillets

DIRECTIONS:

1. Place the first six pesto ingredients into a food processor and blitz until smooth. Place the pesto into a bowl, and add the fish filets, ensuring each one is coated in pesto.

2. Place a griddle pan onto a high heat. Place the pesto-coated fish filets onto the hot griddle pan and grill on both sides until slightly charred, and the fish cooked well but still juicy. Serve the fish with the leftover pesto on top.

NUTRITION: Calories 488 Fat 24 g Carbs 3 g Protein 61.9 g

49. Mussels with Tomatoes & Garlic

Preparation time: 15 minutes

Cooking time: 10 minutes

Servings: 4

INGREDIENTS:

- 4 tbsps. olive oil
- 8 garlic cloves, chopped
- 1 onion, chopped
- 4 cups chopped tomatoes
- 2 tbsps. balsamic vinegar
- 4 lbs./1.8 kg. fresh mussels, debearded and scrubbed
- Salt and pepper
- Large handful freshly chopped parsley

DIRECTIONS:

1. Add the olive oil to a large sauté pan over a medium-high heat. Add the garlic and onions and stir as they become soft and

fragrant. Add the tomatoes and vinegar and allow to simmer for about 5 minutes.

2. Add the mussels, cover the pot, and cook for about 3 minutes, giving the pan a good shake here and there to ensure nothing is sticking. Season with salt and pepper, and serve with fresh parsley.

NUTRITION: Calories 385 Fat 21.3 g Carbs 23.9 g Protein 26.5 g

50. Shrimps & Vegetables Stir-Fry

Preparation time: 15 minutes

Cooking time: 22 minutes

Servings: 4

INGREDIENTS:

- 4 oz. shrimps
- 2 tbsps. olive oil
- 1 onion
- 1 minced garlic clove
- 1 red bell pepper
- 1 green bell pepper
- 1 cup broccoli florets
- 1 cup snow peas
- ½ tsp. salt
- ½ tsp. red pepper flakes
- 1/8 tsp. ground ginger

DIRECTIONS:

1. Wash the shrimps under the cold water. Set aside. Cook broccoli in boiling water for 5-7 minutes. Drain the water and set aside.

2. In a medium-high heat pan, sauté the onion and the garlic in olive oil. Once the onion became translucent, add bell peppers, broccoli, and the snow peas.

3. Stir for 7-10 minutes or until tender over medium-high heat. Add the shrimps and stir for 3-5 minutes until pink. Season with salt, red pepper flakes, and ground ginger.

NUTRITION: Calories 245 Fat 5.7 g Carbs 20 g Protein 30 g

51. Garlic Skillet Salmon

Preparation time: 5 minutes

Cooking time: 14-16 minutes

Servings: 4

INGREDIENTS:

- 1 tablespoon extra-virgin olive oil
- 2 garlic cloves, minced
- 1 teaspoon smoked paprika
- 1½ cups grape or cherry tomatoes, quartered
- 1 (12-ounce / 340-g) jar roasted red peppers, drained and chopped
- 1 tablespoon water
- ¼ teaspoon freshly ground black pepper
- ¼ teaspoon kosher or sea salt

- 1 pound (454 g) salmon fillets, skin removed and cut into 8 pieces
- 1 tablespoon freshly squeezed lemon juice

DIRECTIONS:

1. In a large skillet over medium heat, heat the oil. Add the garlic and smoked paprika and cook for 1 minute, stirring often. Add the tomatoes, roasted peppers, water, black pepper, and salt.

2. Turn up the heat to medium-high, bring to a simmer, and cook for 3 minutes, stirring occasionally and smashing the tomatoes with a wooden spoon toward the end of the cooking time.

3. Add the salmon to the skillet, and spoon some of the sauce over the top. Cover and cook for 10 to 12 minutes, or until the salmon is cooked through and just starts to flake.

4. Remove the skillet from the heat, and drizzle lemon juice over the top of the fish. Stir the sauce, then break up the salmon into chunks with a fork. Serve hot.

NUTRITION: Calories: 255 Fat: 11.7g Protein: 24.2g Carbs: 5.9g

MAIN RECIPES: POULTRY

52. Flavorful Mediterranean Chicken

Preparation Time: 10 minutes

Cooking Time: 20 minutes

Servings: 8

INGREDIENTS:

- 2 lb. chicken thighs
- 1/2 cup olives
- 28 oz can tomato, diced
- 1 1/2 tsp dried oregano
- 2 tsp dried parsley
- 1/2 tsp ground coriander powder
- 1/4 tsp chili pepper
- 1 tsp onion powder
- 1 tsp paprika
- 2 cups onion, chopped
- 2 tbsp olive oil
- Pepper
- Salt

DIRECTIONS:

1. Add oil into the inner pot of instant pot and set the pot on sauté mode. Add chicken and cook until browned. Transfer chicken on a plate. Add onion and sauté for 5 minutes.

2. Add all spices, tomatoes, and salt and cook for 2-3 minutes. Return chicken to the pot and stir everything well. Seal pot with lid and cook on high for 8 minutes.

3. Once done, release pressure using quick release. Remove lid. Add olives and stir well. Serve and enjoy.

NUTRITION: Calories 292 Fat 13 g Carbohydrates 8.9 g Protein 34.3 g

53. Artichoke Olive Chicken

Preparation Time: 10 minutes

Cooking Time: 8 minutes

Servings: 6

INGREDIENTS:

- 2 1/2 lb. chicken breasts, skinless and boneless
- 14 oz can artichokes
- 1/2 cup olives, pitted
- 3/4 cup prunes
- 1 tbsp capers
- 1 1/2 tbsp garlic, chopped
- 3 tbsp red wine vinegar
- 2 tsp dried oregano
- 1/3 cup wine

- Pepper
- Salt

DIRECTIONS:

1. Add all ingredients except chicken into the instant pot and stir well. Add chicken and mix well. Seal pot with lid and cook on high for 8 minutes.

2. Once done, allow to release pressure naturally for 10 minutes then release remaining using quick release. Remove lid. Serve and enjoy.

NUTRITION: Calories 472 Fat 15.5 g Carbohydrates 22.7 g Protein 57.6 g

54. Easy Chicken Piccata

Preparation Time: 10 minutes

Cooking Time: 41 minutes

Servings: 6

INGREDIENTS:

- 8 chicken thighs, bone-in, and skin-on
- 2 tbsp fresh parsley, chopped
- 1 tbsp olive oil
- 3 tbsp capers
- 2 tbsp fresh lemon juice
- 1/2 cup chicken broth
- 1/4 cup dry white wine
- 1 tbsp garlic, minced

DIRECTIONS:

1. Add oil into the inner pot of instant pot and set the pot on sauté mode. Add garlic and sauté for 1 minute. Add wine and cook for 5 minutes or until wine reduced by half.

2. Add lemon juice and broth and stir well. Add chicken and seal pot with the lid and select manual and set a timer for 30 minutes.

3. Once done, release pressure using quick release. Remove lid. Remove chicken from pot and place on a baking tray. Broil chicken for 5 minutes. Add capers and stir well. Garnish with parsley and serve.

NUTRITION: Calories 406 Fat 17 g Carbohydrates 1.2 g Protein 57 g

55. Garlic Thyme Chicken Drumsticks

Preparation Time: 10 minutes

Cooking Time: 18 minutes

Servings: 4

INGREDIENTS:

- 8 chicken drumsticks, skin-on
- 2 tbsp balsamic vinegar
- 2/3 cup can tomato, diced
- 6 garlic cloves
- 1 tsp lemon zest, grated
- 1 tsp dried thyme
- 1/4 tsp red pepper flakes

- 1 1/2 onions, cut into wedges
- 1 tbsp olive oil
- Pepper
- Salt

DIRECTIONS:

1. Add oil into the inner pot of instant pot and set the pot on sauté mode. Add onion and 1/2 tsp salt and sauté for 2-3 minutes.

2. Add chicken, garlic, lemon zest, red pepper flakes, and thyme and mix well. Add vinegar and tomatoes and stir well.

3. Seal pot with lid and cook on high for 15 minutes. Once done, release pressure using quick release. Remove lid. Stir well and serve.

NUTRITION: Calories 220 Fat 8.9 g Carbohydrates 7.8 g Protein 26.4 g

56. Tender Chicken & Mushrooms

Preparation Time: 10 minutes

Cooking Time: 21 minutes

Servings: 6

INGREDIENTS:

- 1 lb. chicken breasts, skinless, boneless, & cut into 1-inch pieces
- 1/4 cup olives, sliced
- 2 oz feta cheese, crumbled
- 1/4 cup sherry
- 1 cup chicken broth

- 1 tsp Italian seasoning

- 12 oz mushrooms, sliced

- 2 celery stalks, diced

- 1 tsp garlic, minced

- 1/2 cup onion, chopped

- 2 tbsp olive oil

- Pepper

- Salt

DIRECTIONS:

1. Add oil into the inner pot of instant pot and set the pot on sauté mode. Add mushrooms, celery, garlic, and onion and sauté for 5-7 minutes.

2. Add chicken, Italian seasoning, pepper, and salt and stir well and cook for 4 minutes. Add sherry and broth and stir well. Seal pot with lid and cook on high for 10 minutes.

3. Once done, allow to release pressure naturally for 10 minutes then release remaining using quick release. Remove lid. Add olives and feta cheese and stir well. Serve and enjoy.

NUTRITION: Calories 244 Fat 13.5 g Carbohydrates 4.1 g Protein 26 g

57. Delicious Chicken Casserole

Preparation Time: 10 minutes

Cooking Time: 20 minutes

Servings: 4

INGREDIENTS:

- 1 lb. chicken breasts, skinless, boneless, & cubed
- 2 tsp paprika
- 3 tbsp tomato paste
- 1 cup chicken stock
- 4 tomatoes, chopped
- 1 small eggplant, chopped
- 1 tbsp Italian seasoning
- 2 bell pepper, sliced
- 1 onion, sliced
- 1 tbsp garlic, minced
- 1 tbsp olive oil
- Pepper
- Salt

DIRECTIONS:

1. Add oil into the inner pot of instant pot and set the pot on sauté mode. Season chicken with pepper and salt and add into the instant pot. Cook chicken until lightly golden brown.

2. Remove chicken from pot and place on a plate. Add garlic and onion and sauté until onion is softened about 3-5 minutes.

3. Return chicken to the pot. Pour remaining ingredients over chicken and stir well. Seal pot with lid and cook on high for 10 minutes.

4. Once done, release pressure using quick release. Remove lid. Stir well and serve.

NUTRITION: Calories 356 Fat 13.9 g Carbohydrates 22.7 g Protein 36.9 g

58. Perfect Chicken & Rice

Preparation Time: 10 minutes

Cooking Time: 25 minutes

Servings: 4

INGREDIENTS:

- 1 lb. chicken breasts, skinless and boneless
- 1 tsp olive oil
- 1 cup onion, diced
- 1 tsp garlic minced
- 4 carrots, peeled and sliced
- 1 tbsp Mediterranean spice mix
- 2 cups brown rice, rinsed
- 2 cups chicken stock
- Pepper
- Salt

DIRECTIONS:

1. Add oil into the inner pot of instant pot and set the pot on sauté mode. Add garlic and onion and sauté until onion is softened.

2. Add stock, carrot, rice, and Mediterranean spice mix and stir well. Place chicken on top of rice mixture and season with pepper and salt. Do not mix.

3. Seal pot with a lid and select manual and set timer for 20 minutes. Once done, allow to release pressure naturally for 10 minutes then release remaining using quick release. Remove lid.

4. Remove chicken from pot and shred using a fork. Return shredded chicken to the pot and stir well. Serve and enjoy.

NUTRITION: Calories 612 Fat 12.4 g Carbohydrates 81.7 g Protein 41.1 g

59. Moroccan Chicken

Preparation Time: 10 minutes

Cooking Time: 25 minutes

Servings: 6

INGREDIENTS:

- 2 lb. chicken breasts, cut into chunks
- 1/2 tsp cinnamon
- 1 tsp turmeric
- 1/2 tsp ginger
- 1 tsp cumin
- 2 tbsp Dijon mustard
- 1 tbsp molasses
- 1 tbsp honey
- 2 tbsp tomato paste
- 5 garlic cloves, chopped
- 2 onions, cut into quarters
- 2 green bell peppers, cut into strips

- 2 red bell peppers, cut into strips
- 2 cups olives, pitted
- 1 lemon, peeled and sliced
- 2 tbsp olive oil
- Pepper
- Salt

DIRECTIONS:

1. Add oil into the inner pot of instant pot and set the pot on sauté mode. Add chicken and sauté for 5 minutes. Add remaining ingredients and stir everything well.

2. Seal pot with a lid and select manual and set timer for 20 minutes. Once done, release pressure using quick release. Remove lid. Stir well and serve.

NUTRITION: Calories 446 Fat 21.2 g Carbohydrates 18.5 g Protein 45.8 g

60. Flavorful Cafe Rio Chicken

Preparation Time: 10 minutes

Cooking Time: 12 minutes

Servings: 6

INGREDIENTS:

- 2 lb. chicken breasts, skinless and boneless
- 1/2 cup chicken stock
- 2 1/2 tbsp ranch seasoning
- 1/2 tbsp ground cumin

- 1/2 tbsp chili powder
- 1/2 tbsp garlic, minced
- 2/3 cup Italian dressing
- Pepper
- Salt

DIRECTIONS:

1. Add chicken into the instant pot. Mix together remaining ingredients and pour over chicken. Seal pot with a lid and select manual and set timer for 12 minutes.

2. Once done, allow to release pressure naturally for 10 minutes then release remaining using quick release. Remove lid. Shred the chicken using a fork and serve.

NUTRITION: Calories 382 Fat 18.9 g Carbohydrates 3.6 g Protein 44.1 g

61. Zesty Veggie Chicken

Preparation Time: 10 minutes

Cooking Time: 5 minutes

Servings: 4

INGREDIENTS:

- 1 lb. chicken tender, skinless, boneless and cut into chunks
- 10 oz of frozen vegetables
- 1/3 cup zesty Italian dressing
- 1/2 tsp Italian seasoning
- 1 cup fried onions

- 2/3 cup rice
- 1 cup chicken broth
- Pepper
- Salt

DIRECTIONS:

1. Add all ingredients except vegetables into the instant pot. Meanwhile, cook frozen vegetables in microwave according to packet instructions.
2. Seal pot with lid and cook on high for 5 minutes. Once done, allow to release pressure naturally for 10 minutes then release remaining using quick release. Remove lid.
3. Add cooked vegetables and stir well. Serve and enjoy.

NUTRITION: Calories 482 Fat 15.9 g Carbohydrates 40.5 g Protein 38.3 g

MAIN RECIPES:

VEGETABLE

62. Healthy Vegetable Medley

Preparation time: 15 minutes

Cooking time: 12 minutes

Servings: 6

INGREDIENTS:

- 3 cups broccoli florets
- 1 sweet potato, chopped
- 1 teaspoon garlic, minced
- 14 oz. coconut milk
- 28 oz. can tomato, chopped
- 14 oz. can chickpeas, drained and rinsed
- 1 onion, chopped
- 1 tablespoon olive oil
- 1 teaspoon Italian seasoning
- Pepper
- Salt

DIRECTIONS:

1. Add oil into the inner pot of instant pot and set the pot on sauté mode. Add garlic and onion and sauté until onion is softened.

2. Add remaining ingredients and stir everything well. Seal pot with lid and cook on high for 12 minutes.

3. Once done, allow to release pressure naturally for 10 minutes then release remaining using quick release. Remove lid.Stir well and serve.

NUTRITION: Calories: 322 Fat: 19.3 g Carbs: 34.3 g Protein: 7.9 g

63. Mediterranean Brussels Sprouts

Preparation time: 15 minutes

Cooking time: 23 minutes

Servings: 4

INGREDIENTS:

- 2 cups Brussels sprouts, cut in half
- ¼ cup feta cheese, crumbled
- ¼ cup olive oil
- 1 bay leaf
- 2 teaspoons pine nuts, roasted
- ½ cup olives
- 2 tablespoons sun-dried tomatoes, chopped
- Pepper
- Salt

DIRECTIONS:

1. Preheat the oven to 3500 F. Heat 1 tablespoon of oil in a pan over medium heat. Add Brussels sprouts and salt and cook for 7-8 minutes. Place pan in oven and bake sprouts of 10 minutes.

2. Meanwhile, in separate pan heat remaining oil over medium heat. Add sun-dried tomatoes and olives and cook for 5 minutes.

3. Remove sprouts from oven and mix with tomato olive mixture. Top with crumbled cheese and pine nuts. Serve and enjoy.

NUTRITION: Calories: 182 Fat: 17.5 g Carbs: 5.9 g Protein: 3.2 g

64. Healthy Garlic Eggplant

Preparation time: 15 minutes

Cooking time: 5 minutes

Servings: 4

INGREDIENTS:

- 1 eggplant, cut into 1-inch pieces
- ½ cup of water
- ¼ cup Can tomato, crushed
- ½ teaspoon Italian seasoning
- 1 teaspoon paprika
- ½ teaspoon chili powder
- 1 teaspoon garlic powder
- 2 tablespoons olive oil
- Salt

DIRECTIONS:

1. Add water and eggplant into the instant pot. Seal pot with lid and cook on high for 5 minutes. Once done, release pressure using quick release. Remove lid.

2. Drain eggplant well and clean the instant pot. Add oil into the inner pot of the instant pot and set the pot on sauté mode.

3. Add eggplant along with remaining ingredients and stir well and cook for 5 minutes. Serve and enjoy.

NUTRITION: Calories: 97 Fat: 7.5 g Carbs: 8.2 g Protein: 1.5 g

65. Indian Bell Peppers and Potato Stir Fry

Preparation time: 15 minutes

Cooking time: 10 minutes

Servings: 2

INGREDIENTS:

- 1 tablespoon oil
- ½ teaspoon cumin seeds
- 4 cloves of garlic, minced
- 4 potatoes, scrubbed and halved
- Salt and pepper to taste
- 5 tablespoons water
- 2 bell peppers, seeded and julienned
- Chopped cilantro for garnish

DIRECTIONS:

1. Heat oil in a skillet over medium flame and toast the cumin seeds until fragrant. Add the garlic until fragrant. Stir in the potatoes, salt, pepper, water, and bell peppers.

2. Close the lid and allow to simmer for at least 10 minutes. Garnish with cilantro before cooking time ends. Place in individual containers.

3. Put a label and store it in the fridge. Allow thawing at room temperature before heating in the microwave oven.

NUTRITION: Calories: 83 Fat: 6.4 g Carbs: 7.3 g Protein: 2.8 g

66. Carrot Potato Medley

Preparation time: 15 minutes

Cooking time: 15 minutes

Servings: 6

INGREDIENTS:

- 4 lbs. baby potatoes, clean and cut in half
- 1 ½ lb. carrots, cut into chunks
- 1 teaspoon Italian seasoning
- 1 ½ cups vegetable broth
- 1 tablespoon garlic, chopped
- 1 onion, chopped
- 2 tablespoons olive oil
- Pepper
- Salt

DIRECTIONS:

1. Add oil into the inner pot of the instant pot and set the pot on sauté mode. Add onion and sauté for 5 minutes. Add carrots and cook for 5 minutes.

2. Add remaining ingredients and stir well. Seal pot with lid and cook on high for 5 minutes.

3. Once done, allow to release pressure naturally for 10 minutes then release remaining using quick release. Remove lid. Stir and serve.

NUTRITION: Calories: 283 Fat: 5.6 g Carbs: 51.3 g Protein: 10.2 g

67. Honey Sweet Potatoes:

Preparation time: 15 minutes

Cooking time: 35 minutes

Servings: 8

INGREDIENTS:

- 4 large sweet potatoes, peel and cut into 1-inch cubes
- ¼ teaspoon paprika
- 2 tablespoons olive oil
- 8 sage leaves
- 1 teaspoon honey
- 2 teaspoons vinegar
- ½ teaspoon of sea salt

DIRECTIONS:

1. Preheat the oven to 3750 F. Add sweet potato, olive oil, sage, and salt in a large bowl and toss well.Roast for 35 minutes.

2. Add honey, vinegar, and paprika and mix well.Serve and enjoy.

NUTRITION: Calories: 90 Fat: 3.5 g Carbs: 14 g Protein: 1 g

68. Flavors Basil Lemon Ratatouille

Preparation time: 15 minutes

Cooking time: 10 minutes

Servings: 8

INGREDIENTS:

- 1 small eggplant, cut into cubes
- 1 cup fresh basil
- 2 cups grape tomatoes
- 1 onion, chopped
- 2 summer squash, sliced
- 2 zucchinis, sliced
- 2 tablespoons vinegar
- 2 tablespoons tomato paste
- 1 tablespoon garlic, minced
- 1 fresh lemon juice
- ¼ cup olive oil
- Salt

DIRECTIONS:

1. Add basil, vinegar, tomato paste, garlic, lemon juice, oil, and salt into the blender and blend until smooth. Add eggplant, tomatoes, onion, squash, and zucchini into the instant pot.

2. Pour blended basil mixture over vegetables and stir well. Seal pot with lid and cook on high for 10 minutes. Once done, allow to release pressure naturally. Remove lid. Stir well and serve.

NUTRITION: Calories: 103 Fat: 6.8 g Carbs: 10.6 g Protein: 2.4 g

69. Roasted Parmesan Cauliflower

Preparation time: 15 minutes

Cooking time: 30 minutes

Servings: 4

INGREDIENTS:

- 8 cups cauliflower florets
- 1 teaspoon dried marjoram
- 2 tablespoons olive oil
- ½ cup parmesan cheese, shredded
- 2 tablespoons vinegar
- ¼ teaspoon pepper
- ¼ teaspoon salt

DIRECTIONS:

1. Preheat the oven to 4500 F. Toss cauliflower, marjoram, oil, pepper, and salt. Toss well. Spread cauliflower onto the baking tray and roast for 15-20 minutes.
2. Toss cauliflower with cheese and vinegar. Return cauliflower to the oven and roast for 5-10 minutes more. Serve and enjoy.

NUTRITION: Calories: 196 Fat: 13 g Carbs: 11 g Protein: 11 g

70. Delicious Pepper Zucchini

Preparation time: 15 minutes

Cooking time: 0 minutes

Servings: 6

INGREDIENTS:

- 1 zucchini, sliced

- 2 poblano peppers, sliced

- 1 tablespoon sour cream

- ½ teaspoon ground cumin

- 1 yellow squash, sliced

- 1 tablespoon garlic, minced

- ½ onion, sliced

- 1 tablespoon olive oil

DIRECTIONS:

1. Add oil into the inner pot of the instant pot and set the pot on sauté mode. Add poblano peppers and sauté for 5 minutes

2. Add onion and garlic and sauté for 3 minutes. Add remaining ingredients except for sour cream and stir well. Seal pot with lid and cook on high for 2 minutes.

3. Once done, release pressure using quick release. Remove lid. Add sour cream and stir well and serve.

NUTRITION: Calories: 42 Fat: 2.9 g Carbs: 4 g Protein: 1 g

71. Brussels Sprouts with Cranberries

Preparation time: 15 minutes

Cooking time: 10 minutes

Servings: 6

INGREDIENTS:

- 1 lb. Brussels sprouts, cut in half

- ½ cup blue cheese, crumbled

- ½ cup dried cranberries
- ½ pecans, toasted
- 1 tablespoon vinegar
- 3 tablespoons olive oil
- Pepper
- Salt

DIRECTIONS:

1. Heat oil in a pan over medium-high heat. Add Brussels sprouts and cook for 5 minutes. Season with pepper and salt and cook for 5 minutes more.

2. Drizzle with vinegar and stir well. Remove pan from heat. Transfer Brussels sprouts to a large bowl and tosses in the cheese, pecans, and cranberries. Serve and enjoy.

NUTRITION: Calories: 170 Fat: 13.8 g Carbs: 8.7 g Protein: 5.5 g

RICE, BEANS, AND GRAINS

RECIPES

72. Baked Brown Rice

Preparation time: 15 minutes

Cooking time: 1 hour & 25 minutes

Servings: 4-6

INGREDIENTS:

- ½ cup minced fresh parsley
- ¾ cup jarred roasted red peppers, rinsed, patted dry, and chopped
- 1 cup chicken or vegetable broth
- 1½ cups long-grain brown rice, rinsed
- 2 onions, chopped fine
- 2¼ cups water
- 4 teaspoons extra-virgin olive oil
- Grated Parmesan cheese
- Lemon wedges
- Salt and pepper

DIRECTIONS:

1. Place the oven rack in the center of the oven and pre-heat your oven to 375 degrees. Heat oil in a Dutch oven on moderate heat until it starts to shimmer.

2. Put in onions and 1 teaspoon salt and cook, stirring intermittently, till they become tender and well browned, 12 to 14 minutes.

3. Mix in water and broth and bring to boil. Mix in rice, cover, and move pot to oven. Bake until rice becomes soft and liquid is absorbed, 65 to 70 minutes.

4. Remove pot from oven. Sprinkle red peppers over rice, cover, and allow to sit for about five minutes.

5. Put in parsley to rice and fluff gently with fork to combine. Sprinkle with salt and pepper to taste. Serve with grated Parmesan and lemon wedges.

NUTRITION: Calories: 100 Carbs: 27g Fat: 21g Protein: 2g

73. Barley Pilaf

Preparation time: 15 minutes

Cooking time: 45 minutes

Servings: 4-6

INGREDIENTS:

- ¼ cup minced fresh parsley
- 1 small onion, chopped fine
- 1½ cups pearl barley, rinsed
- 1½ teaspoons lemon juice
- 1½ teaspoons minced fresh thyme or ½ teaspoon dried

- 2 garlic cloves, minced
- 2 tablespoons minced fresh chives
- 2½ cups water
- 3 tablespoons extra-virgin olive oil
- Salt and pepper

DIRECTIONS:

1. Heat oil in a big saucepan on moderate heat until it starts to shimmer. Put in onion and ½ teaspoon salt and cook till they become tender, approximately 5 minutes.

2. Mix in barley, garlic, and thyme and cook, stirring often, until barley is lightly toasted and aromatic, approximately three minutes.

3. Mix in water and bring to simmer. Decrease heat to low, cover, and simmer until barley becomes soft and water is absorbed, 20 to 40 minutes.

4. Remove from the heat, lay clean dish towel underneath lid and let pilaf sit for about ten minutes. Put in parsley, chives, and lemon juice to pilaf and fluff gently with fork to combine. Sprinkle with salt and pepper to taste. Serve.

NUTRITION: Calories: 39 Carbs: 8g Fat: 1g Protein: 1g

74. Basmati Rice Pilaf Mix

Preparation time: 15 minutes

Cooking time: 25 minutes

Servings: 4-6

INGREDIENTS:

- ¼ cup currants
- ¼ cup sliced almonds, toasted
- ¼ teaspoon ground cinnamon
- ½ teaspoon ground turmeric
- 1 small onion, chopped fine
- 1 tablespoon extra-virgin olive oil
- 1½ cups basmati rice, rinsed
- 2 garlic cloves, minced
- 2¼ cups water
- Salt and pepper

DIRECTIONS:

1. Heat oil in a big saucepan on moderate heat until it starts to shimmer. Put in onion and ¼ teaspoon salt and cook till they become tender, approximately 5 minutes.

2. Put in rice, garlic, turmeric, and cinnamon and cook, stirring often, until grain edges begin to turn translucent, approximately three minutes.

3. Mix in water and bring to simmer. Decrease heat to low, cover, and simmer gently until rice becomes soft and water is absorbed, 16 to 18 minutes.

4. Remove from the heat, drizzle currants over pilaf. Cover, laying clean dish towel underneath lid, and let pilaf sit for about ten minutes.

5. Put in almonds to pilaf and fluff gently with fork to combine. Sprinkle with salt and pepper to taste. Serve.

NUTRITION: Calories: 180 Carbs: 36g Fat: 2g Protein: 4g

75. Brown Rice Salad with Asparagus, Goat Cheese, and Lemon

Preparation time: 15 minutes

Cooking time: 35 minutes

Servings: 4-6

INGREDIENTS:

- ¼ cup minced fresh parsley
- ¼ cup slivered almonds, toasted
- 1 pound asparagus, trimmed and cut into 1-inch lengths
- 1 shallot, minced
- 1 teaspoon grated lemon zest plus 3 tablespoons juice
- 1½ cups long-grain brown rice
- 2 ounces goat cheese, crumbled (½ cup)
- 3½ tablespoons extra-virgin olive oil
- Salt and pepper

DIRECTIONS:

1. Bring 4 quarts water to boil in a Dutch oven. Put in rice and 1½ teaspoons salt and cook, stirring intermittently, until rice is tender, about half an hour.

2. Drain rice, spread onto rimmed baking sheet, and drizzle with 1 tablespoon lemon juice. Allow it to cool completely, about 15 minutes.

3. Heat 1 tablespoon oil in 12-inch frying pan on high heat until just smoking. Put in asparagus, ¼ teaspoon salt, and ¼ teaspoon pepper and cook, stirring intermittently, until asparagus is

browned and crisp-tender, about 4 minutes; move to plate and allow to cool slightly.

4. Beat remaining 2½ tablespoons oil, lemon zest and remaining 2 tablespoons juice, shallot, ½ teaspoon salt, and ½ teaspoon pepper together in a big container.

5. Put in rice, asparagus, 2 tablespoons goat cheese, 3 tablespoons almonds, and 3 tablespoons parsley. Gently toss to combine and allow to sit for about 10 minutes.

6. Sprinkle with salt and pepper to taste. Move to serving platter and drizzle with remaining 2 tablespoons goat cheese, remaining 1 tablespoon almonds, and remaining 1 tablespoon parsley. Serve.

NUTRITION: Calories: 197 Carbs: 6g Fat: 16g Protein: 7g

76. Carrot-Almond-Bulgur Salad

Preparation time: 1 hour & 45 minutes

Cooking time: 0 minutes

Servings: 4-6

INGREDIENTS:

- 1/8 teaspoon cayenne pepper
- 1/3 cup chopped fresh cilantro
- 1/3 cup chopped fresh mint
- 1/3 cup extra-virgin olive oil
- ½ cup sliced almonds, toasted
- ½ teaspoon ground cumin

- 1 cup water

- 1½ cups medium-grind bulgur, rinsed

- 3 scallions, sliced thin

- 4 carrots, peeled and shredded

- 6 tablespoons lemon juice (2 lemons)

- Salt and pepper

DIRECTIONS:

1. Mix bulgur, water, ¼ cup lemon juice, and ¼ teaspoon salt in a container. Cover and allow to sit at room temperature until grains are softened and liquid is fully absorbed, about 1½ hours.

2. Beat remaining 2 tablespoons lemon juice, oil, cumin, cayenne, and ½ teaspoon salt together in a big container.

3. Put in bulgur, carrots, scallions, almonds, mint, and cilantro and gently toss to combine. Sprinkle with salt and pepper to taste. Serve.

NUTRITION: Calories: 240 Carbs: 54g Fat: 2g Protein: 7g

77. Chickpea-Spinach-Bulgur

Preparation time: 15 minutes

Cooking time: 23 minutes

Servings: 4-6

INGREDIENTS:

- ¾ cup chicken or vegetable broth

- ¾ cup water

- 1 (15-ounce) can chickpeas, rinsed

- 1 cup medium-grind bulgur, rinsed
- 1 onion, chopped fine
- 1 tablespoon lemon juice
- 2 tablespoons za'atar
- 3 garlic cloves, minced
- 3 ounces (3 cups) baby spinach, chopped
- 3 tablespoons extra-virgin olive oil
- Salt and pepper

DIRECTIONS:

1. Heat 2 tablespoons oil in a big saucepan on moderate heat until it starts to shimmer. Put in onion and ½ teaspoon salt and cook till they become tender, approximately 5 minutes.

2. Mix in garlic and 1 tablespoon za'atar and cook until aromatic, approximately half a minute. Mix in bulgur, chickpeas, broth, and water and bring to simmer. Decrease heat to low, cover, and simmer gently until bulgur is tender, 16 to 18 minutes.

3. Remove from the heat, lay clean dish towel underneath lid and let bulgur sit for about ten minutes.

4. Put in spinach, lemon juice, remaining 1 tablespoon za'atar, and residual 1 tablespoon oil and fluff gently with fork to combine. Sprinkle with salt and pepper to taste. Serve.

NUTRITION: Calories: 319 Carbs: 43g Fat: 12g Protein: 10g

78. <u>Italian Seafood Risotto</u>

Preparation time: 15 minutes

Cooking time: 60 minutes

Servings: 4-6

INGREDIENTS:

- 1/8 teaspoon saffron threads, crumbled
- 1 (14.5-ounce) can diced tomatoes, drained
- 1 cup dry white wine
- 1 onion, chopped fine
- 1 tablespoon lemon juice
- 1 teaspoon minced fresh thyme or ¼ teaspoon dried
- 12 ounces large shrimp (26 to 30 per pound), peeled and deveined, shells reserved
- 12 ounces small bay scallops
- 2 bay leaves
- 2 cups Arborio rice
- 2 cups chicken broth
- 2 tablespoons minced fresh parsley
- 2½ cups water
- 4 (8-ounce) bottles clam juice
- 5 garlic cloves, minced
- 5 tablespoons extra-virgin olive oil
- Salt and pepper

DIRECTIONS:

1. Bring shrimp shells, broth, water, clam juice, tomatoes, and bay leaves to boil in a big saucepan on moderate to high heat. Decrease the heat to a simmer and cook for 20 minutes.

2. Strain mixture through fine-mesh strainer into big container, pressing on solids to extract as much liquid as possible; discard solids. Return broth to now-empty saucepan, cover, and keep warm on low heat.

3. Heat 2 tablespoons oil in a Dutch oven on moderate heat until it starts to shimmer. Put in onion and cook till they become tender, approximately 5 minutes.

4. Put in rice, garlic, thyme, and saffron and cook, stirring often, until grain edges begin to turn translucent, approximately 3 minutes.

5. Put in wine and cook, stirring often, until fully absorbed, approximately three minutes. Mix in 3½ cups warm broth, bring to simmer, and cook, stirring intermittently, until almost fully absorbed, about 15 minutes.

6. Carry on cooking rice, stirring often and adding warm broth, 1 cup at a time, every few minutes as liquid is absorbed, until rice is creamy and cooked through but still somewhat firm in center, about 15 minutes.

7. Mix in shrimp and scallops and cook, stirring often, until opaque throughout, approximately three minutes. Remove pot from heat, cover, and allow to sit for about 5 minutes.

8. Adjust consistency with remaining warm broth as required. Mix in remaining 3 tablespoons oil, parsley, and lemon juice and sprinkle with salt and pepper to taste. Serve.

NUTRITION: Calories: 450 Carbs: 12g Fat: 40g Protein: 31g

79. Classic Stovetop White Rice

Preparation time: 15 minutes

Cooking time: 22 minutes

Servings: 4-6

INGREDIENTS:

- 1 tablespoon extra-virgin olive oil

- 2 cups long-grain white rice, rinsed

- 3 cups water

- Basmati, jasmine, or Texmati rice can be substituted for the long-grain rice.

- Salt and pepper

DIRECTIONS:

1. Heat oil in a big saucepan on moderate heat until it starts to shimmer. Put in rice and cook, stirring frequently, until grain edges begin to turn translucent, approximately 2 minutes.

2. Put in water and 1 teaspoon salt and bring to simmer. Cover, decrease the heat to low, and simmer gently until rice becomes soft and water is absorbed, approximately 20 minutes.

3. Remove from the heat, lay clean dish towel underneath lid and let rice sit for about ten minutes. Gently fluff rice with fork. Sprinkle with salt and pepper to taste. Serve.

NUTRITION: Calories: 160 Carbs: 36g Fat: 0g Protein: 3g

80. Classic Tabbouleh

Preparation time: 2 hours

Cooking time: 0 minutes

Servings: 4-6

INGREDIENTS:

- 1/8 teaspoon cayenne pepper
- ¼ cup lemon juice (2 lemons)
- ½ cup medium-grind bulgur, rinsed
- ½ cup minced fresh mint
- 1½ cups minced fresh parsley
- 2 scallions, sliced thin
- 3 tomatoes, cored and cut into ½-inch pieces
- 6 tablespoons extra-virgin olive oil
- Salt and pepper

DIRECTIONS:

1. Toss tomatoes with ¼ teaspoon salt using a fine-mesh strainer set over bowl and let drain, tossing occasionally, for 30 minutes; reserve 2 tablespoons drained tomato juice.

2. Toss bulgur with 2 tablespoons lemon juice and reserved tomato juice in a container and allow to sit until grains start to become tender, 30 to 40 minutes.

3. Beat remaining 2 tablespoons lemon juice, oil, cayenne, and ¼ teaspoon salt together in a big container. Put in tomatoes, bulgur, parsley, mint, and scallions and toss gently to combine.

4. Cover and allow to sit at room temperature until flavors have blended and bulgur is tender, about 1 hour. Before serving, toss salad to recombine and sprinkle with salt and pepper to taste.

NUTRITION: Calories: 150 Carbs: 8g Fat: 12g Protein: 4g

81. Farro Cucumber-Mint Salad

Preparation time: 15 minutes

Cooking time: 30 minutes

Servings: 4-6

INGREDIENTS:

- 1 cup baby arugula
- 1 English cucumber, halved along the length, seeded, and cut into ¼-inch pieces
- 1½ cups whole farro
- 2 tablespoons lemon juice
- 2 tablespoons minced shallot
- 2 tablespoons plain Greek yogurt
- 3 tablespoons chopped fresh mint
- 3 tablespoons extra-virgin olive oil
- 6 ounces cherry tomatoes, halved
- Salt and pepper

DIRECTIONS:

1. Bring 4 quarts water to boil in a Dutch oven. Put in farro and 1 tablespoon salt, return to boil, and cook until grains are soft with slight chew, 15 to 30 minutes.

2. Drain farro, spread in rimmed baking sheet, and allow to cool completely, about fifteen minutes.

3. Beat oil, lemon juice, shallot, yogurt, ¼ teaspoon salt, and ¼ teaspoon pepper together in a big container.

4. Put in farro, cucumber, tomatoes, arugula, and mint and toss gently to combine. Sprinkle with salt and pepper to taste. Serve.

NUTRITION: Calories: 97 Carbs: 15g Fat: 4g Protein: 2g

SOUP RECIPES

82. Easy Lemon Chicken Soup

Preparation Time: 10 minutes

Cooking Time: 10 minutes

Servings: 2

INGREDIENTS:

- 1 1/2 lb. chicken breasts, boneless
- 3 cups chicken stock
- 1 tbsp fresh lemon juice
- 1/2 tsp garlic powder
- 1/2 onion, chopped
- Pepper
- Salt

DIRECTIONS:

1. Add all ingredients except lemon juice into the inner pot of instant pot and stir well. Seal pot with lid and cook on high for 10 minutes.

2. Once done, allow to release pressure naturally. Remove lid. Remove chicken from pot and shred using a fork. Return shredded chicken to the pot. Stir in lemon juice and serve.

NUTRITION: Calories 676 Fat 26.2 g Carbohydrates 4.4 g Protein 99.9 g

83. Creamy Chicken Soup

Preparation Time: 10 minutes

Cooking Time: 10 minutes

Serving: 6

INGREDIENTS:

- 2 lb. chicken breast, boneless and cut into chunks
- 8 oz cream cheese
- 2 tbsp taco seasoning 1 cup of salsa
- 2 cups chicken stock
- 28 oz can tomato, diced Salt

DIRECTIONS:

1. Add all ingredients except cream cheese into the instant pot. Seal pot with lid and cook on high pressure 10 for minutes.

2. Once done, allow to release pressure naturally. Remove lid. Remove chicken from pot and shred using a fork. Return shredded chicken to the pot. Add cream cheese and stir well. Serve and enjoy.

NUTRITION: Calories 471 Fat 24.1 g Carbohydrates 19.6 g Protein 43.9 g

84. Garlic Squash Broccoli Soup

Preparation Time: 10 minutes

Cooking Time: 15 minutes

Servings: 4

INGREDIENTS:

- 1 lb. butternut squash, peeled and diced
- 1 lb. broccoli florets
- 1 tsp dried basil
- 1 tsp paprika
- 1/2 cups vegetable stock
- 1 tsp garlic, minced
- 1 tbsp olive oil
- 1 onion, chopped Salt

DIRECTIONS:

1. Add oil into the inner pot of instant pot and set the pot on sauté mode. Add onion and garlic and sauté for 3 minutes. Add remaining ingredients and stir well.

2. Seal pot with lid and cook on high pressure 12 for minutes. Once done, allow to release pressure naturally for 10 minutes then release remaining using quick release. Remove lid.

3. Blend soup using an immersion blender until smooth. Serve and enjoy.

NUTRITION: Calories 137 Fat 4.1 g Carbohydrates 24.5 g Protein 5 g

85. Chicken Rice Soup

Preparation Time: 10 minutes

Cooking Time: 9 minutes

Servings: 4

INGREDIENTS:

- 1 lb. chicken breast, boneless

- 2 thyme sprigs
- 1 tsp garlic, chopped
- 1/4 tsp turmeric
- 1 tbsp olive oil
- 1 tbsp fresh parsley, chopped
- 2 tbsp fresh lemon juice
- 1/4 cup rice
- 1/2 cup celery, diced
- 1/2 cup onion, chopped
- 2 carrots, chopped
- 2 cups vegetable stock
- Pepper
- Salt

DIRECTIONS:

1. Add oil into the inner pot of instant pot and set the pot on sauté mode. Add garlic, onion, carrots, and celery and sauté for 3 minutes.
2. Add the rest of the ingredients and stir well. Seal pot with lid and cook on high for 6 minutes.
3. Once done, release pressure using quick release. Remove lid. Shred chicken using a fork. Serve and enjoy.

NUTRITION: Calories 237 Fat 6.8 g Carbohydrates 16.6 g Protein 26.2 g

86. Sausage Potato Soup

Preparation Time: 10 minutes

Cooking Time: 20 minutes

Servings: 6

INGREDIENTS:

- 1 lb. Italian sausage, crumbled
- 1 cup half and half
- 1 cup kale, chopped
- 6 cups chicken stock
- 1/2 tsp dried oregano
- 3 potatoes, peeled and diced
- 1 tsp garlic, minced
- 1 onion, chopped
- 1 tbsp olive oil
- Pepper
- Salt

DIRECTIONS:

1. Add oil into the inner pot of instant pot and set the pot on sauté mode. Add sausage, garlic, and onion and sauté for 5 minutes.
2. Add the rest of the ingredients and stir well. Seal pot with lid and cook on high for 15 minutes.
3. Once done, allow to release pressure naturally for 10 minutes then release remaining using quick release. Remove lid. Stir and serve.

NUTRITION: Calories 426 Fat 29.1 g Carbohydrates 22.3 g Protein 18.9 g

87. Italian Salsa Chicken Soup

Preparation Time: 10 minutes
Cooking Time: 25 minutes
Servings: 6
INGREDIENTS:

- 1 lb. chicken breasts, boneless and cut into chunks
- 3 cups chicken stock
- 8 oz cream cheese
- 1 1/2 cups salsa
- 1 tsp Italian seasoning
- 1 tbsp fresh parsley, chopped
- Pepper
- Salt

DIRECTIONS:

1. Add all ingredients except cream cheese and parsley into the instant pot and stir well. Seal pot with lid and cook on high for 25 minutes.
2. Once done, release pressure using quick release. Remove lid. Remove chicken from pot and shred using a fork. Return shredded chicken to the pot.
3. Add cream cheese and stir well and cook on sauté mode until cheese is melted. Serve and enjoy.

NUTRITION: Calories 301 Fat 19.4 g Carbohydrates 5.6 g Protein 26.1 g

88. Roasted Tomatoes Soup

Preparation Time: 10 minutes

Cooking Time: 5 minutes

Servings: 2

INGREDIENTS:

- 14 oz can fire-roasted tomatoes
- 1 1/2 cups vegetable stock
- 1/4 cup zucchini, grated
- 1/2 tsp dried oregano
- 1/2 tsp dried basil
- 1/2 cup heavy cream
- 1/2 cup parmesan cheese, grated
- 1 cup cheddar cheese, grated
- Pepper
- Salt

DIRECTIONS:

1. Add tomatoes, stock, zucchini, oregano, basil, pepper, and salt into the instant pot and stir well. Seal pot with lid and cook on high for 5 minutes.

2. Once done, release pressure using quick release. Remove lid. Set pot on sauté mode. Add heavy cream, parmesan cheese, and

cheddar cheese and stir well and cook until cheese is melted. Serve and enjoy.

NUTRITION: Calories 460 Fat 34.8 g Carbohydrates 13.5 g Protein 24.1 g

89. Mussels Soup

Preparation Time: 10 minutes

Cooking Time: 3 minutes

Servings: 2

INGREDIENTS:

- 1 ½ pounds mussels, cleaned
- 2 tsp Italian seasoning
- 2 tbsp olive oil
- 1 cup grape tomatoes, chopped
- 4 cups chicken stock
- 1/4 cup fish sauce

DIRECTIONS:

1. Add all ingredients into the inner pot of instant pot and stir well. Seal pot with lid and cook on high for 3 minutes.
2. Once done, release pressure using quick release. Remove lid. Stir well and serve.

NUTRITION: Calories 256 Fat 18.6 g Carbohydrates 9.9 g Protein 14.1 g

90. Healthy Cabbage Soup

Preparation Time: 10 minutes

Cooking Time: 15 minutes

Servings: 4

INGREDIENTS:

- 1 cabbage head, shredded
- 4 cups vegetable stock
- 1/4 cup fresh parsley, chopped
- 1 tbsp garlic, minced
- 1 tbsp olive oil
- 1 onion, chopped
- 1/2 lb. carrots, sliced
- Pepper
- Salt

DIRECTIONS:

1. Add oil into the inner pot of instant pot and set the pot on sauté mode. Add onion and garlic and sauté for 5 minutes.
2. Add the rest of the ingredients and stir well. Seal pot with lid and cook on high for 10 minutes.
3. Once done, allow to release pressure naturally for 10 minutes then release remaining using quick release. Remove lid. Stir and serve.

NUTRITION: Calories 149 Fat 7.4 g Carbohydrates 20.4 g Protein 3.7 g

91. Creamy Carrot Tomato Soup

Preparation Time: 10 minutes

Cooking Time: 10 minutes

Servings: 6

INGREDIENTS:

- 1 can tomatoes, diced
- 1/2 cup heavy cream
- 1 cup vegetable broth
- 1 tbsp dried basil
- 1 onion, chopped
- 4 large carrots, peeled and chopped
- 1/4 cup olive oil
- Pepper Salt

DIRECTIONS:

1. Add oil into the inner pot of instant pot and set the pot on sauté mode. Add onion and carrots and sauté for 5 minutes.

2. Add the rest of ingredients except heavy cream and stir well. Seal pot with lid and cook on high pressure 5 for minutes.

3. Once done, allow to release pressure naturally. Remove lid. Stir in heavy cream and blend soup using an immersion blender until smooth. Serve and enjoy.

NUTRITION: Calories 144 Fat 12.4 g Carbohydrates 7.8 g Protein 1.8 g

DESSERT RECIPES

92. Mediterranean Tomato Salad with Feta and Fresh Herbs

Preparation Time: 10 minutes

Cooking Time: 15 minutes

Servings: 2

INGREDIENTS:

- Diced tomatoes, 5
- Crumbled feta cheese, 2 oz.
- Chopped fresh dill, ½ cup
- Diced onion, ½ cup
- Chopped mint leaves, 6
- Paprika, ½ tsp.
- Olive oil, 3 tbsp.
- Minced garlic, 2 tbsp.
- Lemon juice, 2 tsp.
- White wine vinegar, 2 tsp.
- Salt and black pepper, to taste

DIRECTIONS:

1. Combine the onions, tomatoes, herbs and the garlic in a bowl, then season with your spices (salt, black pepper, paprika).

2. To create the dressing, in a separate bowl first mix together the olive oil, vinegar, and lemon juice.

3. Top with feta cheese

NUTRITION: Calories: 125, Protein: 2 g, Carbohydrates: 8 g, Fat: 9g

93. Quinoa Bowl with Yogurt, Dates, And Almonds

Preparation Time: 10 minutes

Cooking Time: 15 minutes

Servings: 2

INGREDIENTS:

- 1½ cups water
- 1 cup quinoa
- 2 cinnamon sticks
- 1-inch knob of ginger, peeled
- ¼ teaspoon kosher salt
- 1 cup plain Greek yogurt
- ½ cup dates, pitted and chopped
- ½ cup almonds (raw or roasted), chopped
- 2 teaspoons honey (optional)

DIRECTIONS:

1. Bring the water, quinoa, cinnamon sticks, ginger, and salt to a boil in a medium saucepan over high heat.

2. Reduce the heat to a simmer and cover; simmer for 10 to 12 minutes. Remove the cinnamon sticks and ginger. Fluff with a fork.

3. Add the yogurt, dates, and almonds to the quinoa and mix together. Divide evenly among 4 bowls and garnish with ½ teaspoon honey per bowl, if desired.

4. Use any nuts or seeds you like in place of the almonds.

NUTRITION: Calories: 125, Protein: 2 g, Carbohydrates: 8 g, Fat: 9g

94. Almond Butter Banana Chocolate Smoothie

Preparation Time: 5 minutes

Cooking Time: 30 minutes

Servings: 2

INGREDIENTS:

- ¾ cup almond milk
- ½ medium banana, preferably frozen
- ¼ cup frozen blueberries
- 1 tablespoon almond butter
- 1 tablespoon unsweetened cocoa powder
- 1 tablespoon chia seeds

DIRECTIONS:

1. In a blender or Vitamix, add all the ingredients. Blend to combine.

2. Peanut butter, sunflower seed butter, and other nut butters are good choices to replace the almond butter

NUTRITION: Calories: 125, Protein: 2 g, Carbohydrates: 8 g, Fat: 9g

95. Strawberry Rhubarb Smoothie

Preparation Time: 8 minutes

Cooking Time: 0 minutes

Servings: 2

INGREDIENTS:

- 1 Cup Strawberries, Fresh & Sliced
- 1 Rhubarb Stalk, Chopped
- 2 Tablespoons Honey, Raw
- 3 Ice Cubes
- 1/8 Teaspoon Ground Cinnamon
- ½ Cup Greek Yogurt, Plain

DIRECTIONS:

1. Start by getting out a small saucepan and fill it with water. Place it over high heat to bring it to a boil, and then add in your rhubarb.
2. Boil for three minutes before draining and transferring it to a blender.
3. In your blender add in your yogurt, honey, cinnamon and strawberries. Blend until smooth, and then add in your ice.
4. Blend until there are no lumps and it's thick. Enjoy cold.

NUTRITION: Calories: 295, Protein: 6 g, Fat: 8 g, Carbs: 56 g

96. Walnut & Date Smoothie

Preparation Time: 10 minutes

Cooking Time: 0 minutes

Servings: 2

INGREDIENTS:

- 4 Dates, Pitted
- ½ Cup Milk
- 2 Cups Greek Yogurt, Plain
- 1/2 Cup Walnuts
- ½ Teaspoon Cinnamon, Ground
- ½ Teaspoon Vanilla Extract, Pure
- 2-3 Ice Cubes

DIRECTIONS:

1. Blend everything together until smooth, and then serve chilled.

NUTRITION: Calories: 385, Protein: 21 g, Fat: 17 g, Carbs: 35 g

97. Vanilla Apple Compote

Preparation Time: 10 minutes

Cooking Time: 15 minutes

Servings: 2

INGREDIENTS:

- 3 cups apples, cored and cubed
- 1 tsp. vanilla
- 3/4 cup coconut sugar

- 1 cup of water
- 2 tbsp. fresh lime juice

DIRECTIONS:

2. Add all ingredients into the inner pot of instant pot and stir well.
3. Seal pot with lid and cook on high for 15 minutes.
4. Once done, allow to release pressure naturally for 10 minutes then release remaining using quick release. Remove lid.
5. Stir and serve.

NUTRITION: Calories 76 Fat 0.2 g Carbohydrates 19.1 g Sugar 11.9 g Protein 0.5 g Cholesterol 0 mg

98. Apple Dates Mix

Preparation Time: 10 minutes

Cooking Time: 15 minutes

Servings: 2

INGREDIENTS:

- 4 apples, cored and cut into chunks
- 1 tsp. vanilla
- 1 tsp. cinnamon
- 1/2 cup dates, pitted
- 1 1/2 cups apple juice

DIRECTIONS:

1. Add all ingredients into the inner pot of instant pot and stir well.
2. Seal pot with lid and cook on high for 15 minutes.

3. Once done, allow to release pressure naturally for 10 minutes then release remaining using quick release. Remove lid.

4. Stir and serve.

NUTRITION: Calories 226 Fat 0.6 g Carbohydrates 58.6 g Sugar 46.4 g Protein 1.3 g Cholesterol 0 mg

99. Lemon Pear Compote

Preparation Time: 10 minutes

Cooking Time: 15 minutes

Servings: 2

INGREDIENTS:

- 3 cups pears, cored and cut into chunks
- 1 tsp. vanilla
- 1 tsp. liquid stevia
- 1 tbsp. lemon zest, grated
- 2 tbsp. lemon juice

DIRECTIONS:

1. Add all ingredients into the inner pot of instant pot and stir well.

2. Seal pot with lid and cook on high for 15 minutes.

3. Once done, allow to release pressure naturally for 10 minutes then release remaining using quick release. Remove lid.

4. Stir and serve.

NUTRITION: Calories 50 Fat 0.2 g Carbohydrates 12.7 g Sugar 8.1 g Protein 0.4 g Cholesterol 0 mg

100. Strawberry Stew

Preparation Time: 10 minutes

Cooking Time: 15 minutes

Servings: 2

INGREDIENTS:

- 12 oz. fresh strawberries, sliced
- 1 tsp. vanilla
- 1 1/2 cups water
- 1 tsp. liquid stevia
- 2 tbsp. lime juice

DIRECTIONS:

1. Add all ingredients into the inner pot of instant pot and stir well.
2. Seal pot with lid and cook on high for 15 minutes.
3. Once done, allow to release pressure naturally for 10 minutes then release remaining using quick release. Remove lid.
4. Stir and serve.

NUTRITION: Calories 36 Fat 0.3 g Carbohydrates 8.5 g Sugar 4.7 g Protein 0.7 g Cholesterol 0 mg

101. Oat and Fruit Parfait

Preparation Time: 10 minutes

Cooking Time: 10 minutes

Servings: 2

INGREDIENTS:

- 1/2 cup whole-grain rolled or quick cooking oats (not instant)

- 1/2 cup walnut pieces

- 1 teaspoon honey

- 1 cup sliced fresh strawberries

- 11/2 cups (12 ounces) vanilla low-fat Greek yogurt

- Fresh mint leaves for garnish

DIRECTIONS:

1. Preheat the oven to 300°F.

2. Spread the oats and walnuts in a single layer on a baking sheet

3. Toast the oats and nuts just until you begin to smell the nuts, 10 to 12 minutes. Remove the pan from the oven and set aside.

4. In a small microwave-safe bowl, heat the honey just until warm, about 30 seconds. Add the strawberries and stir to coat.

5. Place 1 tablespoon of the strawberries in the bottom of each of 2 dessert dishes or 8-ounce glasses.

6. Add a portion of yogurt and then a portion of oats and repeat the layers until the containers are full, ending with the berries. Serve immediately or chill until ready to eat.

NUTRITION: Calories: 385, Protein: 21 g, Fat: 17 g, Carbs: 35 g

CONCLUSION

Thank you again for purchasing this book.

As we end, let us leave you with some tips to live a life with Mediterranean Diet.

Spice Things Up with Fresh Herbs and Spices

Fresh herbs and spices are what make most of the recipes insanely delicious, while also providing health benefits. If you already use these in your daily cooking, more power to you! If not, we got you covered!

Consume Seafood Weekly

As we've talked before, one benefit of living close to the sea is easy to access to seafood. However, seafood holds a lower priority than plant-based foods in the Mediterranean diet and should be consumed in moderation. If you're a vegetarian, consider taking fish oil supplements to get those omega-3 fatty acids into your system. Better yet, considering shunning your vegetarianism, and eating seafood to get the vital nourishment only seafood can provide.

Consume Meat Monthly

Red meat used to be a luxury for the Mediterranean people back in the day. Although not completely off-limits, you should try and reduce your red-meat intake as much as possible. If you love red meat, consider consuming it no more than two times per month. And even when you do eat it, make sure the serving size of the meat in the dish is small (two to three-ounce serving). The main reason to limit meat intake is to limit the number of unhealthy fats going into your system. As we talked before, saturated fats and omega-6 fatty acids are not good for health, but unfortunately, red meat contains significant quantities of these. As a beef lover myself, I eat a two-ounce serving of it per month, and when I do eat it, I make sure there are lots of vegetables on the side to satiate my hunger.

Drink Wine!

Love wine? Well, it is your lucky day. Having a glass of wine with dinner is a common practice in the Mediterranean regions. Red wine is especially good for the heart and it is a good idea to consume a glass of red wine twice a week. Excess of everything is bad, and wine is no exception so keep it in check. Also, if you're already suffering from health conditions, it is a good idea to check with your doctor before introducing wine to your daily diet.

Work Your Body

Now you don't have to hit the gym like a maniac to work your body. Walking to your destination instead of driving, taking the stairs instead of the lift, or kneading your dough can all get the job done. So, be creative and work your body when you can. Better yet, play a sport or just hit the gym like a maniac. You don't have to, as I said at the start, but it will help… a lot.

Enjoy a Big Lunch

Lunch was usually the meal of the day when the Mediterranean residents sat with their families and took their time enjoying a big meal. This strengthens social bonds and relaxes the mind during the most stressful time of the day, when you're just halfway done with your work, probably.

Have Fun with Friends and Family

Just spending a few minutes per day doing something fun with your loved ones is great for de-stressing. Today, we don't understand the importance of this, and people feel lonely, and in some cases, even depressed. Just doing this one thing has the power to solve a huge chunk of the problems our modern society faces.

Be Passionate

The Mediterranean people are passionate folk. Living on or close to sun-kissed coasts, their passion for life is naturally high. Being passionate about something in life can take you a long way towards health and wellness.

That will be all, till our next book.